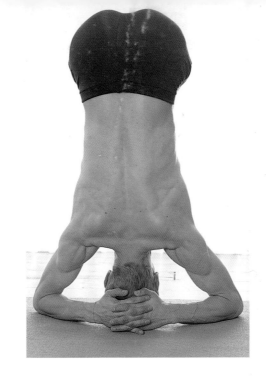

THE PILATES BACK BOOK

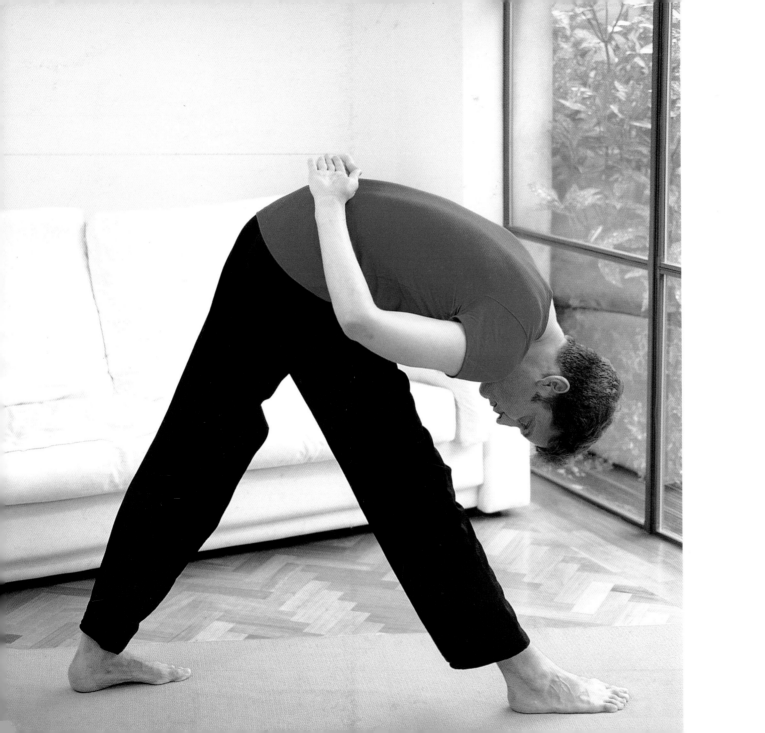

THE PILATES BACK BOOK

Heal Neck, Back, and Shoulder
Pain with Easy Pilates Stretches

FAIR WINDS

P R E S S

Tia Stanmore

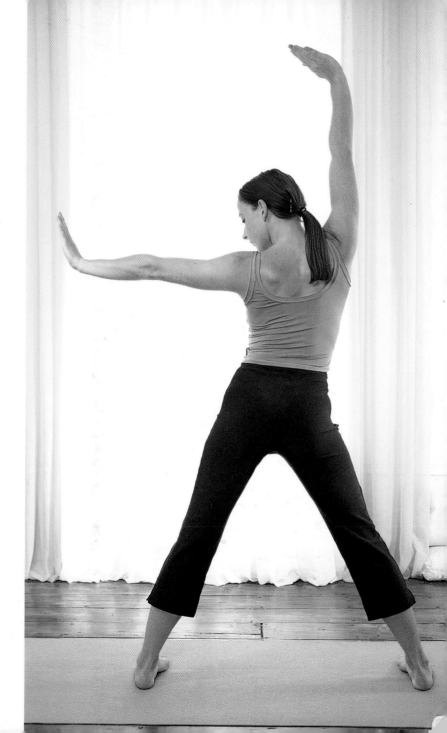

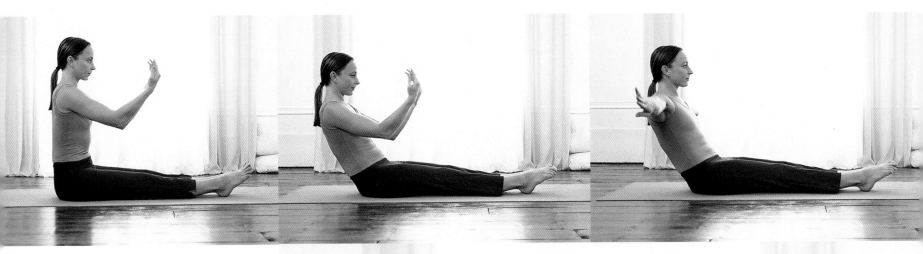

First published in 2002 under the title SPINE WORK by
Hamlyn, a division of Octopus Publishing Group Ltd,
2–4 Heron Quays, London E14 4JP

First published in North America in 2002
under the title THE PILATES BACK BOOK by
Fair Winds Press,
33 Commercial Street,
Gloucester, MA 01930

613.7 71881
STAN

ISBN 1-931412-89-8

A CIP catalogue record for this book is available from the
British Library

Printed and bound in China

10 9 8 7 6 5 4

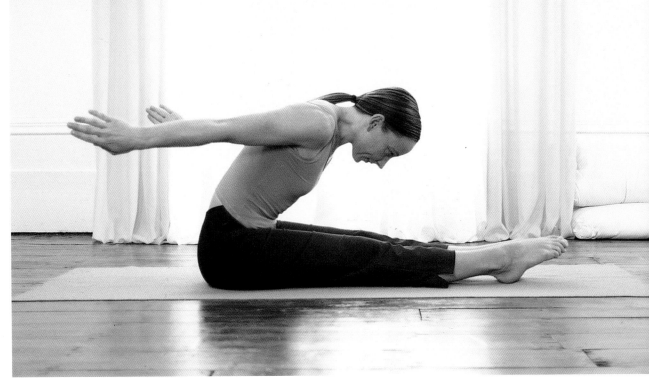

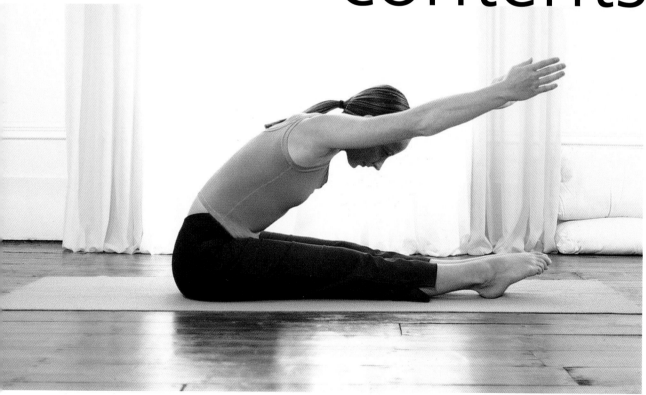

contents

introduction 6

Pilates defined 8

principles and aims of Pilates 10

how Pilates works 12

performing the exercises 14

Pilates and your body 16

the spine 18

movement of the lumbar spine 22

the musculoskeletal system 24

looking after your spine 26

spinal stability 28

Pilates-based programme for the spine 32

preparation 34

how to use this book 36

getting started 38

fundamentals 40

developing strength 61

creating flexibility 101

specialized programmes 115

lumbo-pelvic programme 116

shoulder girdle/upper torso programme 120

glossary 124

index 126

acknowledgements 128

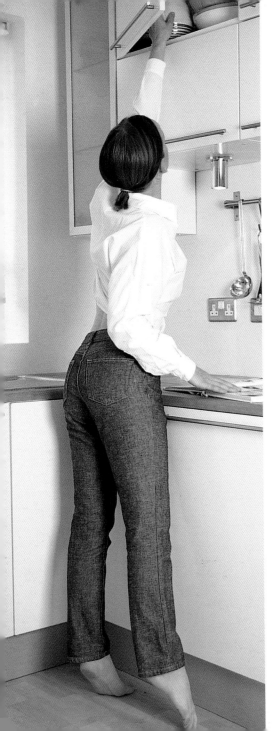

introduction

Movement is fundamental to our existence. As we move through space and time we engage in a wide range of activities in all sorts of different environments, and to do this we need a complex range of skills just to remain upright against the force of gravity. As we go about our daily lives – sitting at a computer, driving a car, carrying a child, running along a beach – our brains process sensory information about where we are in space and the subtleties of our surroundings, and control our muscles accordingly. All of this takes place at a subconscious level, and we are able to make the necessary movements to do the things we want to do without having to focus on our physical self.

Convenient though this is, it is not always good for the health of our bodies. For example, if you sit at a desk for hours, after some time your body will become tired, with stiffness in the joints and tension in the muscles. If this happens on a regular basis and becomes an established pattern, it can have long-term effects that can be detrimental to both the skeletal and muscular systems. It may even cause injuries to the spine.

It takes sustained effort to change subconscious patterns of movement to improve health and posture, and we cannot do it on a conscious level alone. We must replace the repeated harmful patterns of movement with others that do not harm the body. This takes time, and involves changing how we move and developing a greater awareness of the body and how it functions. The overall effect will be to improve the efficiency of the body and allow us to experience life with a greater sense of ourselves and our connection with the environment, and with a greater appreciation of our body and its ability.

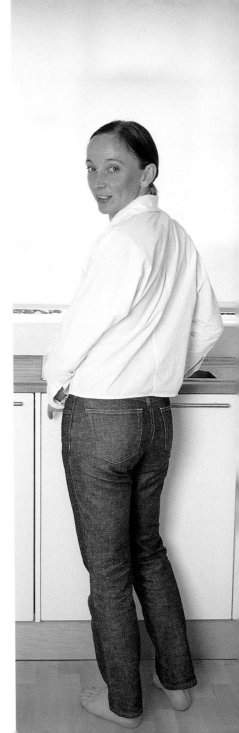

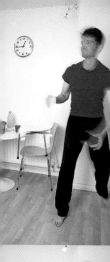

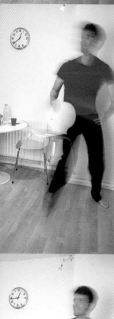

the Pilates-based programme for the spine

The Pilates-based programme for the spine promotes flexibility and strength, as well as stability for the spine; creates a body that is supple and strong; and will teach you how the muscles function to support and protect the spine. It is based on physical therapy, movement analysis, dance and yoga, and can be adapted for all levels of fitness, age ranges and body types. The techniques used are designed to strengthen the abdominal and spinal muscles to help prevent back pain. For those who already suffer from spinal pain, the programme can help to improve posture and movement to prevent its recurrence. It can be beneficial for those with a sedentary lifestyle, those aiming to improve their skill at various sports, and for professional athletes and dancers.

The Pilates system is designed to condition the whole body. It encourages integration of the mind and body, and will help you to achieve precision in muscle control, coordination and fluidity of movement. The programme aims to combine traditional principles of science with complementary disciplines to create an innovative, effective and safe training system.

I hope this book will show you how to correct imbalances in your posture, and also inspire you to explore some or all of the related disciplines further, increasing your knowledge of your body and its functions, and the relationship of body and mind.

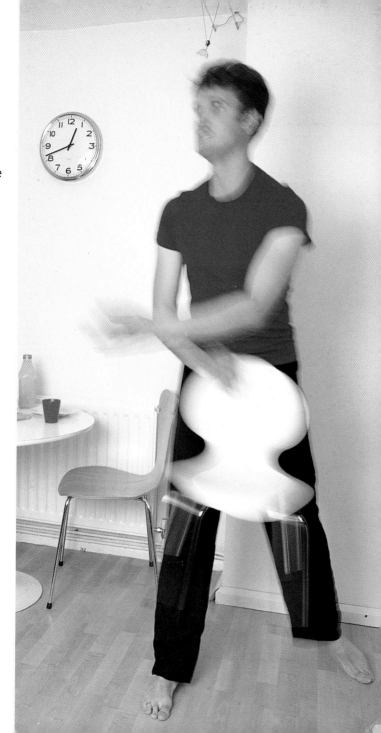

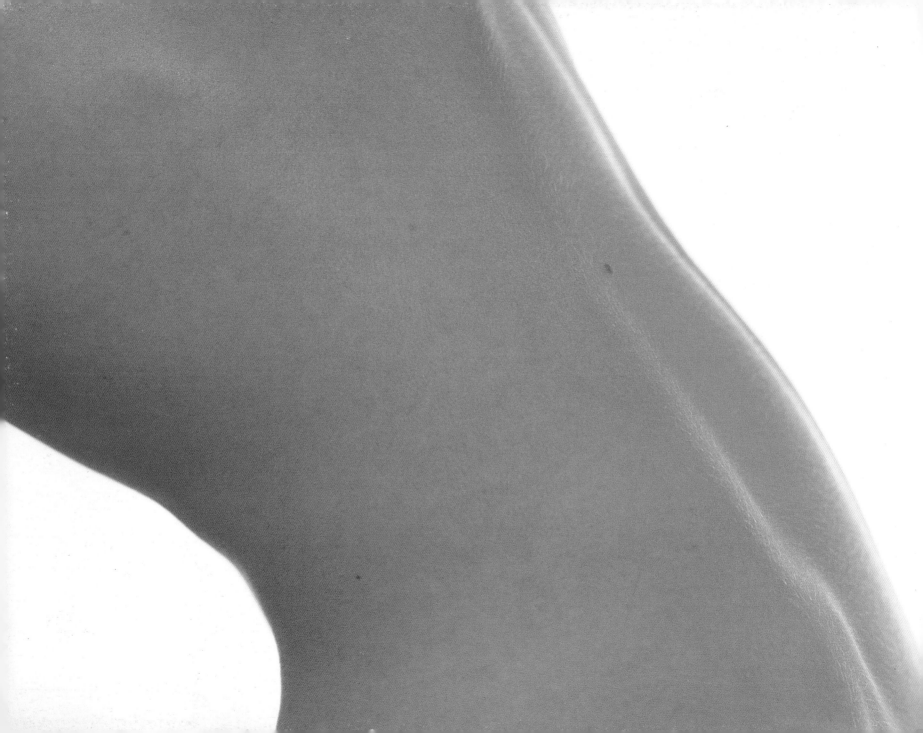

Pilates
defined

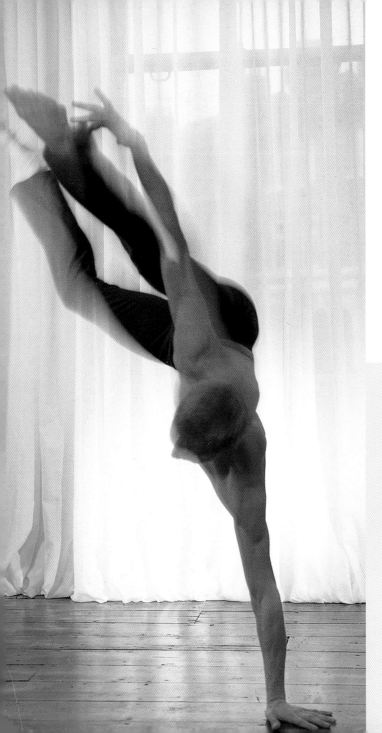

principles and aims of Pilates

The Pilates system, developed by Joseph Pilates in the early 1900s, integrates principles of both Eastern and Western disciplines. Pilates, who described his technique as a method of physical and mental conditioning, was influenced by therapeutic exercise, yoga, dance and martial arts. In the 1920s, he established a studio in New York, where he worked closely with the dance community.

With increased research into human movement and exercise therapy, the system has developed into a number of different forms, but it still largely relies on the perspective and movement patterns of Joseph Pilates' revolutionary work. In recent years, leaders in the field of spinal research have promoted the principles of Pilates in the management of spinal pain, in particular acute and chronic back pain.

Pilates can be beneficial in the management of:

- spinal pain
- soft-tissue injuries
- joint restriction
- injury prevention
- sports injuries
- dance injuries
- occupational overuse syndrome
- antenatal and postnatal care

the aims of Pilates are:

Relaxation – to work without excessive muscle tension and release muscular holding patterns.

Concentration – to perform each exercise with precision and to train the muscles to work automatically.

Alignment – to re-educate the posture and balance of the muscles that surround the joints.

Coordination – to refine the brain's control of the body's movement and dynamic function.

Breathing – to allow the release of any stiffness in the spine and help to control movement.

Flowing movements – to focus on lengthening from the centre of the body and performing movements slowly and smoothly.

Centring – with all exercises, the deep abdominal and spinal muscles work effectively together to stabilize the spine and maintain lumbo-pelvic (lower back) control.

Endurance – to develop the stabilization muscles and integrate them into activities of everyday living, work and sport.

Imaging – to develop an internalized visual sense of the body in both postural alignment and functional movement, which enhances the quality and efficiency of movement.

Integration – to develop a sense of performing all movement with the whole body to balance the effort of the body's muscular and skeletal systems.

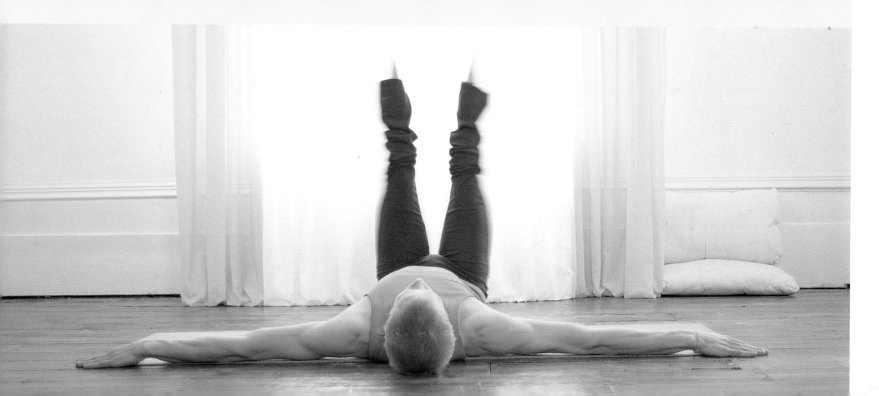

how Pilates works

Pilates is a total body-conditioning system that integrates the mind and body to improve precision in muscle control, strength and flexibility. Pilates achieves quality of movement and function by creating body awareness, coordination and endurance.

The exercises focus on developing the strength of the torso through appropriate use of the spinal muscles, which act as stabilizers and create a vital support for the spine. Performed slowly, with an awareness of the body in movement, the exercises control the body and focus the mind. Breathing, correct initiation of muscle action and postural support are emphasized in every sequence, so the principles may also be applied while carrying out everyday activities.

Pilates develops proximal stability – that is control of the torso without putting stress on the spine, so that all movements are controlled against a stable background. In addition, it can correct any muscle imbalances caused by injury and postural problems by aligning the body correctly and balancing the muscular and external forces acting on the joints and musculoskeletal structures.

If specific movement patterns are repeated regularly it can result in overactivity of some muscle groups and underactivity of others – for example, endurance-type muscles in various exercise regimens, sports and performing arts. This can also happen with recreational activities or in the work environment. For example, a person who lifts regularly using the muscles in the arms and shoulders without the aid of the powerful torso muscles will develop a weakness of the stabilizers – essentially the back and abdominal muscles – as well as weakness and tension in the arm and shoulder muscles. This will eventually cause injury to and degeneration of the unsupported spine. The rest of the body may then compensate for this weakness, which can lead to further injury to other parts of the body. Continued misuse of the musculoskeletal system can spiral into a complicated cycle, but it is preventable and reversible in all but the most extreme cases.

Pilates can form an integral part of rehabilitation from overuse or misuse of the body, reducing the chance of imbalances recurring after recovery. It develops muscles through their full range of motion in various movement patterns, and results in lengthened, flexible muscles with greater strength.

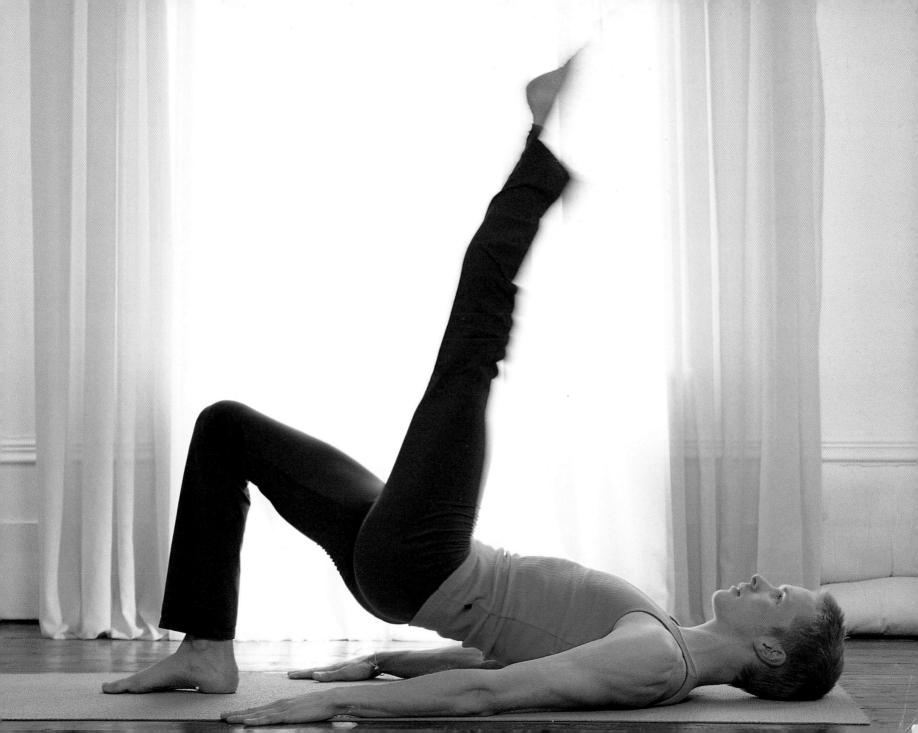

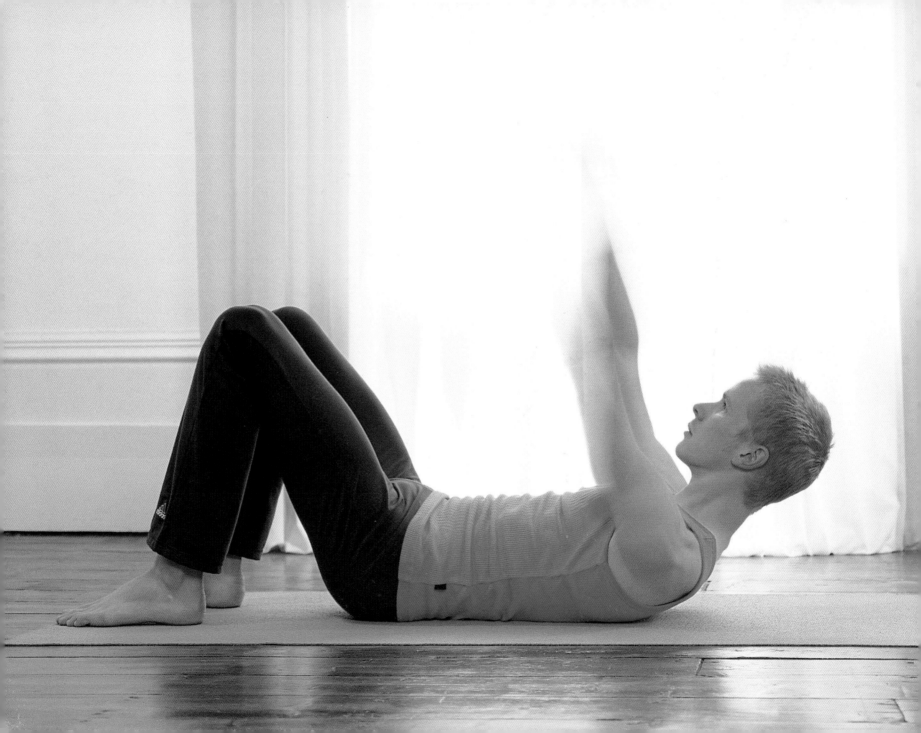

performing
the exercises

To begin with, you should perform the exercises while lying down, so your body is supported. This will allow your body to be in proper alignment as you make each movement. Later, you can perform the exercises in sitting, kneeling and standing positions, and you should integrate the principles into everyday activities. Ultimately, the physical knowledge you derive from the programme will change the way you move and the way in which you perform practical skills, as well as showing you how to refine your body movements in situations that can cause injury. There are two modes fundamental to the Pilates system – mat work and studio work.

mat work

Mat work involves a series of exercises performed in lying, sitting or standing positions. The exercises coordinate strength and postural control, and involve working the muscles of the whole body. The exercises become more challenging as awareness, strength, flexibility, coordination and endurance develop. Mat work forms the basis for the more complex studio work, which in turn trains the body to function at its optimum level.

studio work

A studio class can be either one-to-one or a small group, with instruction based on an individualized programme with specific goals. The exercises involve the use of specialized equipment that works against the body's resistance and resistance provided by springs, which can be adjusted to varying tensions. A pulley system provides further exercise options.

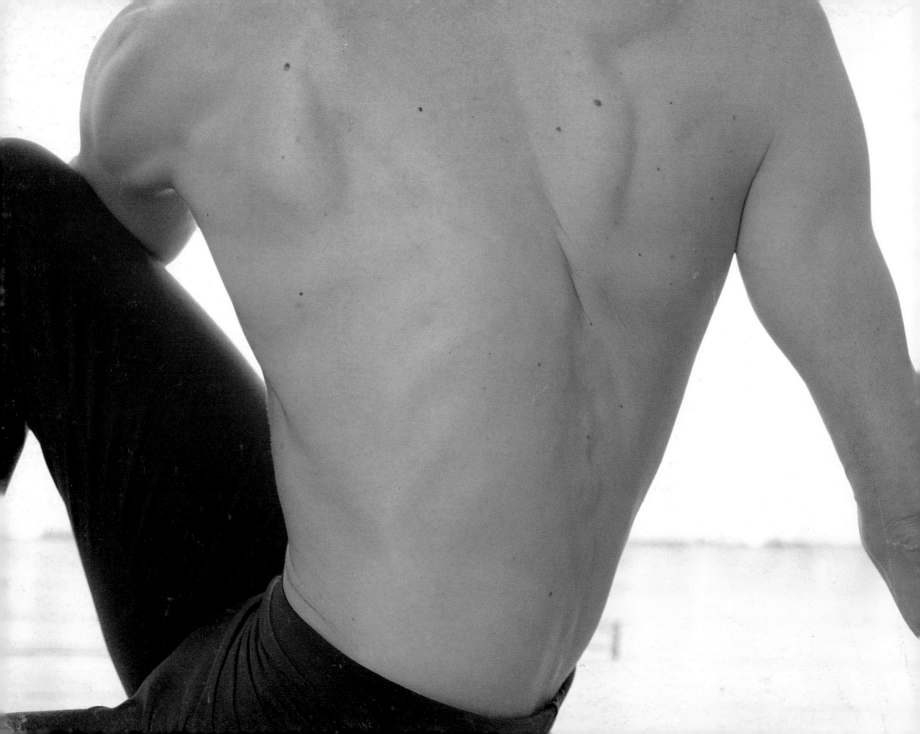

Pilates
and your body

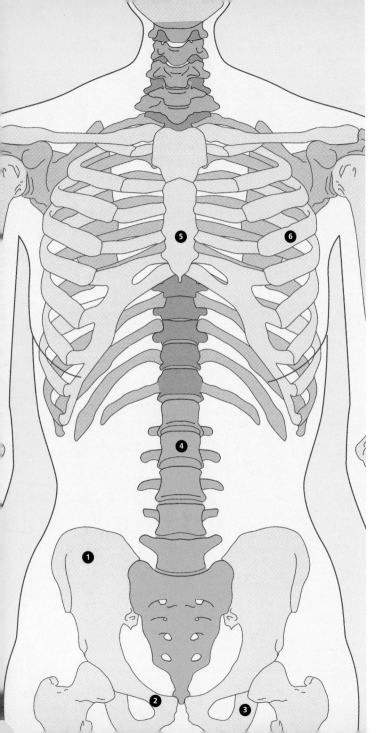

1 Ilium
2 Pubis
3 Ischium
4 Vertebral column
5 Sternum
6 Ribs

the spine

The spine, or backbone, extends from the base of the skull to the base of the pelvis and is made up of 33 separate bones called vertebrae, which surround and protect the spinal cord. The vertebrae are linked by strong ligaments and have flexible discs, called intervertebral discs, positioned between them to act as shock absorbers. The spine is divided into five regions.

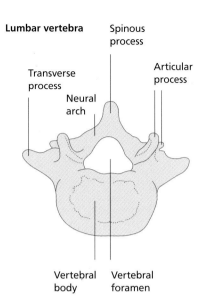

Lumbar vertebra

Spinous process

Transverse process

Articular process

Neural arch

Vertebral body

Vertebral foramen

the vertebrae

A typical vertebra has a body, a neural arch and seven processes – a spinous process, two transverse processes and four articular processes. The vertebral body forms the main part of each vertebra, and it is the vertebral bodies that are linked together to form the spinal column. The body is roughly cylindrical with flattened upper and lower surfaces, which form joints with the adjacent vertebrae through the intervertebral discs. The neural arch surrounds a canal called the vertebral foramen, and the spinal cord runs through this canal. The processes are attached to the neural arch. However, the vertebrae are not identical to each other. The size and shape of each reflects the function it performs according to its position in the spinal column.

the cervical region

The first and uppermost of the spine's five regions is the cervical region. This is the neck region and it is made up of seven vertebrae. The first two vertebrae are specialized to support the head and allow it to move freely.

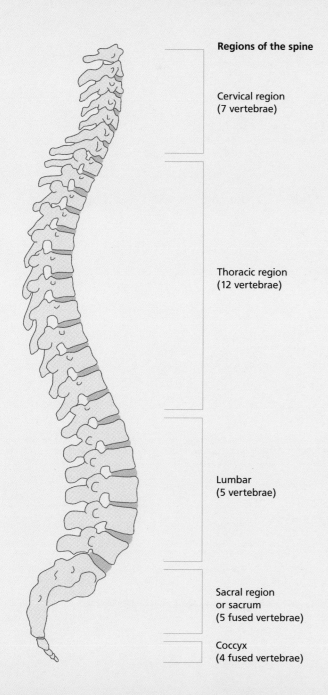

Regions of the spine

Cervical region
(7 vertebrae)

Thoracic region
(12 vertebrae)

Lumbar
(5 vertebrae)

Sacral region
or sacrum
(5 fused vertebrae)

Coccyx
(4 fused vertebrae)

the thoracic region

The thoracic region, or thorax, is the part of the body enclosed by the ribs, and this region of the spine is made up of 12 vertebrae. These vertebrae have special indentations for the ribs on the sides of their bodies and their transverse processes. The thoracic cage is formed from the 12 thoracic vertebrae, the sternum (breastbone) and the 12 pairs of ribs. It changes in volume during breathing as the diaphragm (a dome-shaped muscle lying at the bottom of the lungs), the sternum and the ribs move up and down, increasing as you breathe in and decreasing as you breathe out.

the lumbar region

This region in the small of the back is made up of five vertebrae, which are larger and stronger than the other vertebrae, because they have to support much more load. The lowest lumbar vertebra rests on top of the sacrum.

the sacral region

The sacrum consists of five fused vertebrae. It is positioned at the base of the spine and plays a vital role in supporting the lumbar spine. Forces through the lumbar spine are transmitted to the sacrum and on to the legs.

The sacrum, with the two hip bones (each made up of the ilium, ischium and pubis) and the coccyx, forms the pelvic girdle (or pelvis). This ring of bone links the torso and the lower limbs. It has a diverse range of functions, among them to provide an attachment for muscles, and to support body weight when sitting and standing. The two sacro-iliac joints, where the sacrum meets the ilia, have strong ligaments, which hold the joints steady and absorb the forces placed on them.

the coccyx

The coccyx forms a small appendix to the sacrum. It consists of four vertebrae at the base of the spine, which are usually fused together, although the first may be a separate piece.

spinal joints and the intervertebral discs

There are three joints between each of the vertebrae of the lumbar spine. The intervertebral discs, which are positioned between two adjacent vertebral bodies, form one joint. They have a fibrous outer part (the annulus fibrosus) and a soft fluid central part (the nucleus pulposus). The discs are tied to the ligaments in front of and behind the vertebral bodies and attached to the cartilage that covers the flat upper and lower surfaces of the vertebral bodies, and they cannot move freely. The articular processes form joints on the left and right sides of the vertebra, and these are called the zygapophyseal or facet joints. Each intervertebral disc makes movement between the vertebral segments possible and it acts like a shock absorber. When a force is applied to the disc, the disc absorbs some of that force but also cushions the impact of it on the adjacent vertebrae. The zygapophyseal joints hold the intervertebral joint in place and stop it from being twisted too much or displaced forward.

ligaments

All the joints in all the regions of the spine are bound by ligaments, which limit their movement in certain directions. The whole vertebral column is bonded by two long ligaments. The anterior longitudinal ligament is attached to the fronts of the vertebral bodies and discs from the base of the skull to the top of the sacrum. The posterior ligament is indirectly linked to the base of the skull and passes down behind the vertebral bodies and discs from the second cervical vertebra to the sacrum. The anterior ligament protects the vertebrae from excessive backward movement when the body bends backwards, and the posterior ligament prevents excessive separation of the vertebral bodies when you bend forwards.

1 Intervertebral discs
2 Facet joint
3 Spinal nerve
4 Vertebral processes
5 Vertebral body

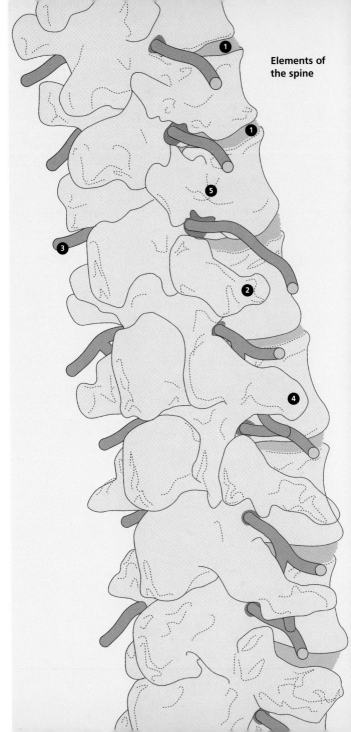

Elements of the spine

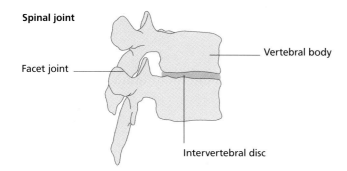

Spinal joint

Facet joint

Vertebral body

Intervertebral disc

lumbar lordosis

In the normal standing position, the lumbar spine has a natural concave curve, known as the lumbar lordosis. The spine consists of a series of curves, each designed for a different function, which develop in relation to gravity. The lumbar lordosis is designed for strength, and is able to absorb forces and transmit weight. It develops when a baby begins to extend its legs and take weight through them. The lumbar spine is positioned above and supported by the sacrum, the upper surface of which is inclined downwards and forwards, so the curve of the lumbar spine keeps the body upright. The lumbar lordosis and a similar curve in the cervical region, the cervical lordosis, are fundamental for maintaining the spine's flexibility and strength. Flattening the back or over-arching the spine, as in the condition hyperlordosis, can cause injury to and early degeneration of the spine.

vertebral canal

The series of holes running through the centre of the vertebrae forms the vertebral foramen or 'canal', which encloses and protects the spinal cord. In the condition called spinal stenosis, the canal becomes narrower, which can put pressure on the spinal nerves. This problem tends to occur in the lumbar region only.

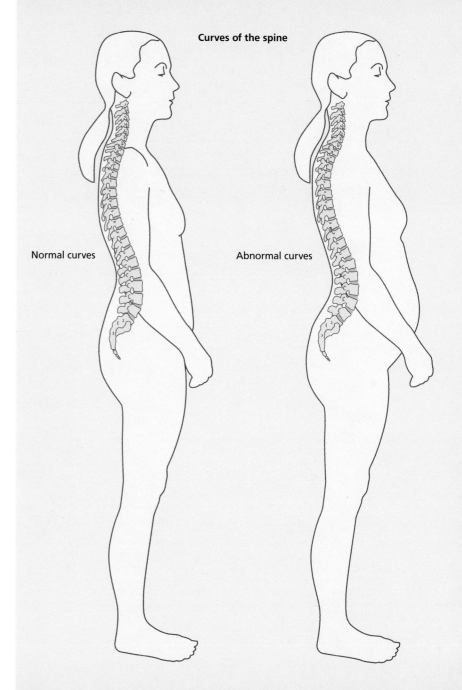

Curves of the spine

Normal curves

Abnormal curves

lumbar movement

The healthy spine is capable of a good range of movement along its entire length. Muscles and ligaments change the position of the vertebrae, while the intervertebral discs absorb shock and give the spine flexibility.

The lumbar spine is capable of a greater range of movement than the thoracic spine because its intervertebral discs are thicker. The outside of the disc has rows of fibrous tissue that can stretch and then return to normal. They function as ligaments, so that whichever way the joint is moved there will always be some fibres that prevent excessive movement.

flexion

Flexion, or bending, of the lumbar region reduces lumbar lordosis, and can take place extremely freely. It is controlled by the spinal muscles, and restricted by the tension of the intervertebral discs and the posterior longitudinal ligament. The tautness of this ligament allows an increase in forward flexibility of the lower lumbar area. However, bending

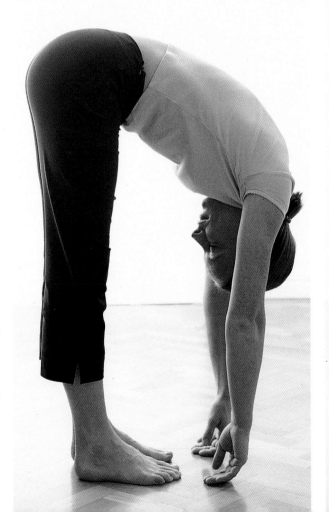

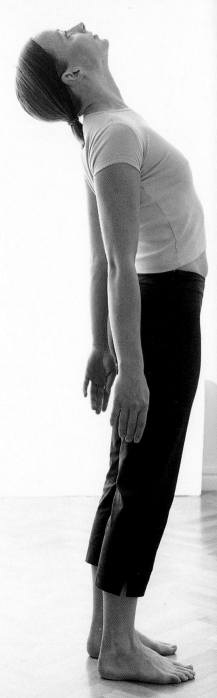

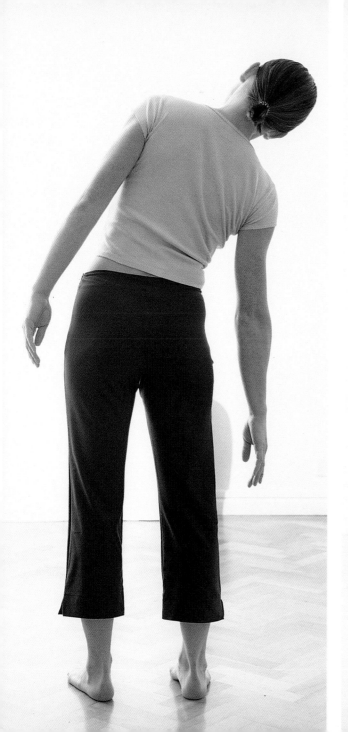

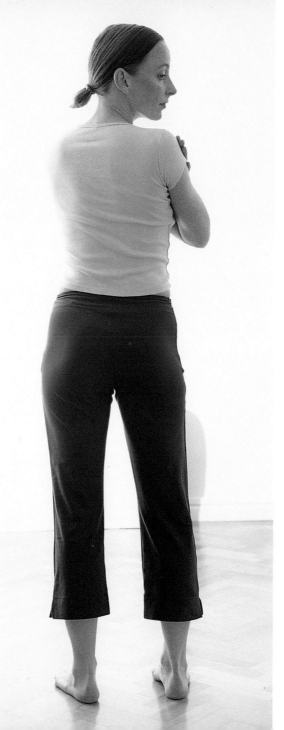

forwards compresses the joint and weakens the posterior support at the sides of the intervertebral discs. This can cause herniation of the discs, where the outer fibrous layer ruptures and some of the soft interior is pushed out.

extension

Extension, or straightening, enhances the lordosis and is controlled by the anterior longitudinal ligament, the intervertebral discs, the large spinous processes and the 'closing' of the zygapophyseal joints.

other movements in the lumbar spine

lateral flexion

Lateral flexion, or sideways bending, of the lumbar spine is highly variable between individuals and it changes with age. By middle age, the range of lateral flexion is about half what it was in childhood.

rotation

The lumbar spine has a minimal range of rotation, or turning. In extension, no rotation is possible because of the position of the zygapophyseal joints. Conversely, as flexion increases so the range of rotation increases.

the musculoskeletal system

The muscular system is involved in producing movement both of the body as a whole and of the internal organs. In the musculoskeletal system, the muscles pull on tendons that are attached to bones to generate movement. Most movements involve more than one group of muscles, and there are hundreds of muscles in the body that can be consciously controlled. Pilates is concerned with movements of the spine, and it is useful to know the muscles that are involved in the various movements and what each one does.

1 Biceps – the main muscle of the front of the upper arm. It bends the elbow and helps to bend and steady the shoulder joint.

2 Triceps – the only muscle at the back of the upper arm. It extends the elbow.

3 Deltoid – encloses the shoulder and the upper arm. It is used to move the arm backwards and forwards.

4 Serratus anterior – links the upper ribs to the scapula (shoulder blade). It draws the shoulder forwards and rotates the scapula.

5 Trapezius – runs down the back of the neck and along the shoulders. It is used to extend the head.

6 Rhomboid – runs between the scapula and the thoracic vertebrae. Most of it lies beneath the trapezius muscle. It is used to brace the shoulder and rotate the scapula.

7 Latissimus dorsi – popularly referred to as 'lats', it runs from the lower chest to the

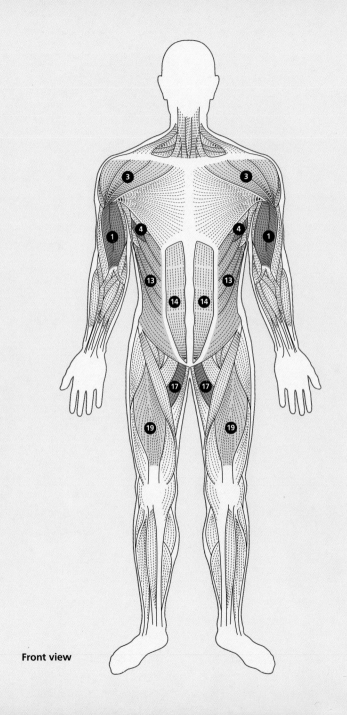

Front view

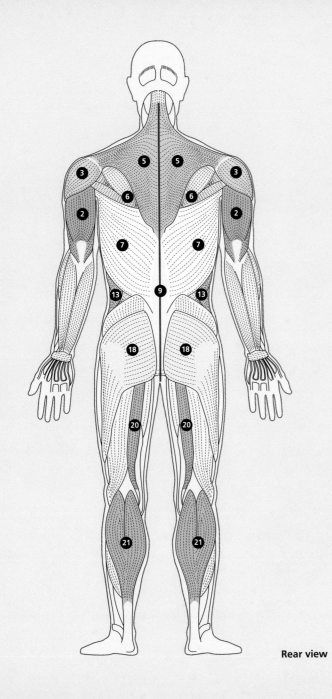

Rear view

lumbar region. It draws the arm backwards, pulls the shoulder down and back and the body upwards.

8 Erector spinae (not shown) – found at the back of the neck, chest and abdomen. This important muscle extends the spine and holds the body upright. When it acts on one side only it bends the spine to that side.

9 Lumbar multifidus – links the lumbar and sacral vertebra in a specialized arrangement of vertebra-to-vertebra attachments. It has a mainly postural function, rather than causing larger movements. Contraction of both sides together extends the torso and neck, and of one side only bends the torso and neck to that side and rotates them.

10 Quadratus lumborum (not shown) – deep interior waist muscle. It helps to extend the spine against a resistance, but its main functions are to bend the torso sideways and stabilize the twelfth 'floating' rib as you breathe in and out.

11 Transversus abdominus (not shown) – deep internal muscle that runs across the abdomen. It applies pressure to the abdomen and holds the organs in place. It lies beneath the internal oblique muscle.

12 Internal oblique (not shown) – crosses the abdomen horizontally. It compresses the abdomen and moves the torso. It lies beneath the external oblique muscle.

13 External oblique – side muscle of the abdomen. It compresses the abdomen and is used when moving the torso in any direction.

14 Rectus abdominis – popularly known as the 'abs', this muscle runs vertically down the entire front of the abdomen. It supports the abdominal organs and draws the front of the pelvis upwards.

15 Coccygeus and levator ani (not shown) – these muscles form the pelvic floor.

16 Psoas (not shown) – also known as the hip flexor. This is a deep muscle that runs from the front of the femur (thigh bone) to the lumbar region of the spine. It acts to bring the thigh forwards at the hip.

17 Adductor – an inner thigh muscle that draws the leg inwards.

18 Gluteus maximus – forms the buttocks. It is important for maintaining the upright posture of the torso on the legs, standing, walking, running and jumping.

19 Quadriceps – runs down the middle of the front of the thigh. It has the opposite action to the semitendinosus.

20 Semitendinosus – also known as the hamstrings. It runs down the middle of the back of the thigh and is used to extend the thigh and flex the knee.

21 Gastrocnemius – forms the greater part of the calf. This muscle runs down the back of the lower leg and gives the force when walking and running.

Pilates and your body

25

looking after your spine

Inappropriate movements can cause spinal injuries and, combined with a lack of awareness of the body's structure and function, can have a cumulative damaging effect. The bones and joints start to degenerate, and the muscles become weak and lose their flexibility. Most of these problems are caused by the bones and muscles that affect the spinal joints and their motion not being properly aligned.

Many lumbar spine injuries are the result of damage to the transversus abdominus and lumbar multifidus muscles, both of which play an important role in maintaining spinal stability and optimum alignment. Leg injuries and reduced flexibility of the hamstrings and gluteal muscles can also cause lumbar spine problems. The postural changes that occur following injury, and the effect these changes have on the way you move, can lead to secondary changes in other areas of the spine, including the thoracic spine, where the ribs attach, and the cervical spine, or neck.

Whether the body is stationary or moving, the alignment of the spine – optimum or otherwise – is constant. For example, someone with a curved spine will maintain this curve whether they are walking or

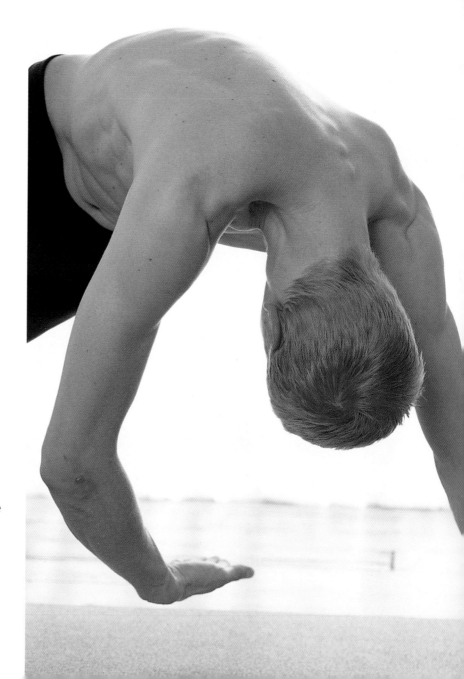

lying down. Conversely, someone with good posture, who moves efficiently and with good quality of movement – without undue tension or excessive muscular effort – will stand or sit with optimum alignment. When the body and the mind become aware of an inefficiency, they will compensate in some very sophisticated ways, for example by pushing out the chest to counterbalance rounding of the upper spine. Unfortunately, this effort will often cause another, less desirable, pattern of movement to develop elsewhere, which can lead to further injury.

An approach to treatment that looks at a muscle or joint or the structure of the body in isolation, without reference to the whole body, will not deal with the problem successfully. Pilates, however, in conjunction with treatment, is highly effective in alleviating and preventing a wide range of spinal and other musculo-skeletal disorders. It is effective because it considers both postural changes and inefficient movement patterns to be causes of pain and disorder. Pilates acknowledges the relationship between the mind, the nervous system and the musculoskeletal system in human function. In essence, it can cause lasting change within the body by accessing the central nervous system (the brain and spinal cord). The brain reprogrammes movement and function to free the body of pain and associated symptoms. Treatment alone will relieve symptoms, but unless the body, directed by the mind, can bring about a permanent change in its function, the symptoms will return. Achieving such a change requires a high level of body awareness and self-knowledge.

therapeutic exercise and pain management

It is possible to correct inefficient ways of functioning and misalignment of the body, and promote movement with efficiency and awareness, by in-depth exploration of movement and the way the body works. Help from an experienced Pilates practitioner skilled in movement analysis and neuromuscular re-education can make this easier to achieve.

But before a practitioner can develop an individual programme of therapeutic exercises to aid recovery, correct dysfunction or help with the prevention of pain, it is essential that he or she has an understanding of the individual's neuromuscular system and patterns of movement. Not only does the practitioner need to have high levels of skill and experience in movement analysis, but also the client must be actively involved – commitment to practice and the integration of new movement patterns and functional activity are basic requirements for bringing about changes in the body.

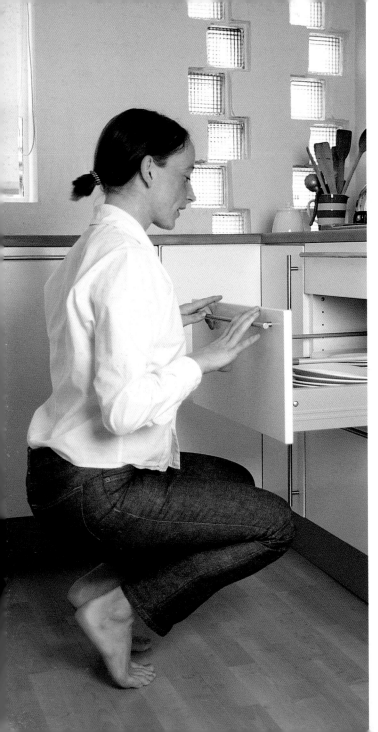

spinal stability

There is a direct connection between reduced spinal stability and spinal pain. Spinal stability is directly influenced by three things: the spinal ligaments and skeletal structure; the muscular system; and the control of the muscular system by the central nervous system. Damage to the muscular system or a failure in the way the muscles are activated by the nervous system, combined with deficiencies in the skeletal structures and ligaments, may cause spinal instability and lead to spinal pain.

The muscles, ligaments and bones, and nervous system are interlinked, and each one is able to compensate in some way for deficiencies in the others. But if there is a problem in one of the three systems and the other systems fail to compensate, this will eventually lead to injury and spinal pain. The stability of the spine also relies on it being able to withstand external and internal forces, and compression of the joints.

The lumbar region is capable of an extremely complex range of movements, and this makes it difficult to maintain control of optimal movement at all times. Each of the lumbar vertebrae needs to be correctly positioned in relation to those above and below and the neuromuscular system must be highly developed.

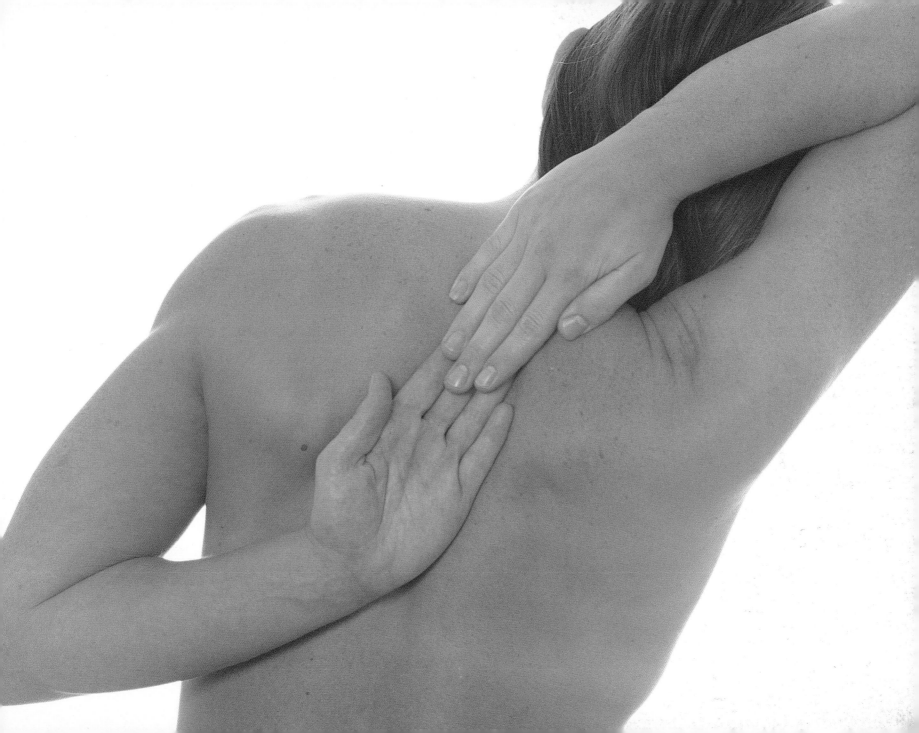

the role of muscles

Spinal stability relies heavily on the muscle system, which compensates for instability by increasing the resistance of the lumbar spine. Tiredness, degeneration and injury can all disrupt normal muscle function, which may lead to spinal instability. Both the torso and the pelvic muscles play a role in stabilization of the spinal joints.

The deep muscles, which include the transversus abdominus and lumbar multifidus, control the relationship between each of the lumbar vertebrae and lumbar spine posture. They provide spinal stability in all activities – whether 'low-load', such as sitting, or highly skilled, such as running – and are fundamental in preventing spinal pain. If you repeatedly overload the spine and its associated structures over a long period of time without involving the deep muscles, the spine will become unstable and painful.

The larger muscles of the trunk, which include the latissimus dorsi, serratus anterior and trapezius, are involved in spinal movement as they transfer load between the thorax and the pelvis. These muscles deal with variations in external loads during functional movements so that the resulting load on the spine is reduced.

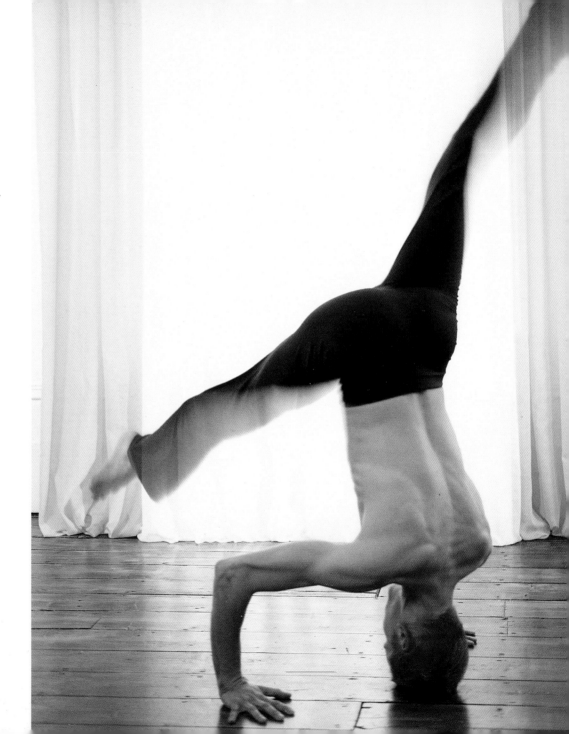

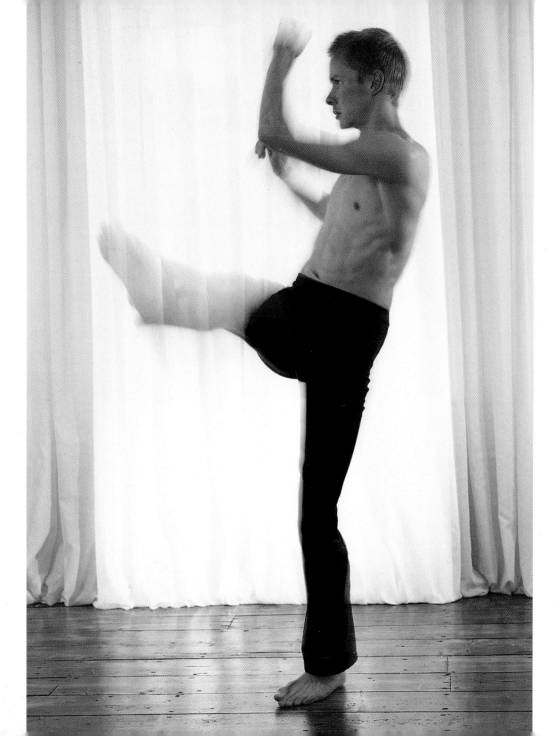

reducing forces on the spine

The deep muscles must stabilize the individual segments of the spine in both sustained postures, for example standing or sitting in the same position for a period of time, and dynamic movement. To maximize their stabilizing role, the forces applied to the lumbar spine must be reduced. This involves creating safe working environments, paying particular attention to posture; adopting safe lifting techniques; and reducing joint forces, which can damage the spine.

Neuromuscular control plays an important role in coordinating the activity of the deep muscles, and it may be the most important element in maintaining spinal stability and preventing spinal pain. It is also important to strengthen and improve the endurance capacity of the larger muscles of the trunk during loading activities, such as lifting heavy loads, as this will reduce the forces that are transferred to the spine and the demands on the deep muscle system.

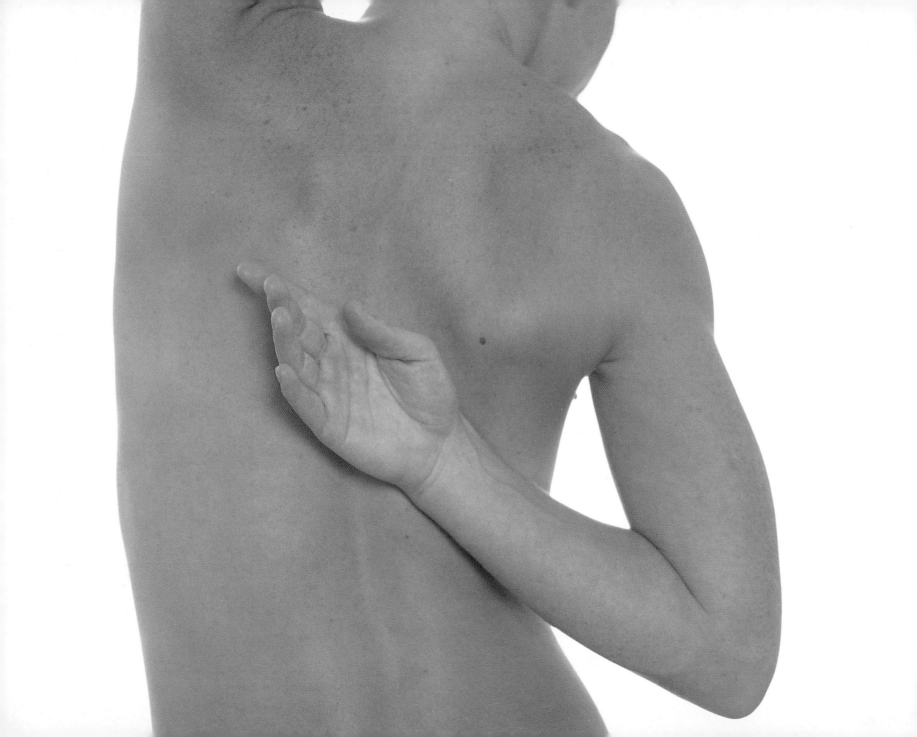

Pilates-based programme
for the spine

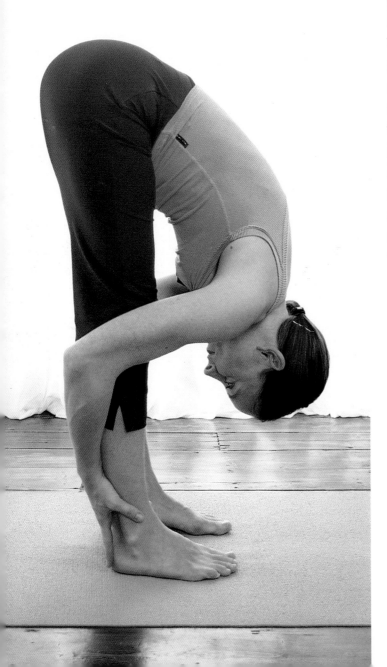

preparation

With any new form of exercise or stretching, it is best to take things slowly at first, as this will allow the body to adapt gradually and in such a way that the effects are immediately beneficial. Developing the skills of listening to your body, gaining an awareness of how you move, and recognizing your strengths and limitations will help you to understand your own physicality, without the risk of injury or misuse of the body.

Initially, you may find you cannot perform the exercises or stretches in full; this may be because you do not have the flexibility to attain an alignment of the spine, or the strength to hold certain postures. With time and commitment, however, the gradual changes to your body will allow you to progress.

To create a body that has quality and efficiency of movement requires intricate balancing of strength and flexibility. To do this, you need first to gain a clear understanding of the fundamentals, which will form the foundations for the more dynamic and challenging exercises. Once you are familiar with the fundamentals, the Pilates-based programme will enable you to have control over how you use your body, thereby minimizing the risk of injury.

practising the programme

The most challenging part of any exercise programme is starting it in the first place! You then have to stick with it and do it on a regular basis, so that the benefits you gain are not lost because of a break in your routine. Medical research has shown that both muscular strength and flexibility decline within a very short space of time once you stop regular exercise and stretching, regardless of your physical fitness level.

Allocate a regular period of time each day to practise the programme; it is a good idea to make this early in the morning, before the rest of your commitments take over. The Pilates-based programme for the spine is designed so you can do it wherever you are – at home, as part of your gym routine or while travelling. You can also adapt the programme to focus on certain areas, such as the lower spine or upper body, or you can perform an extended programme for the whole body, depending on your goals and time constraints.

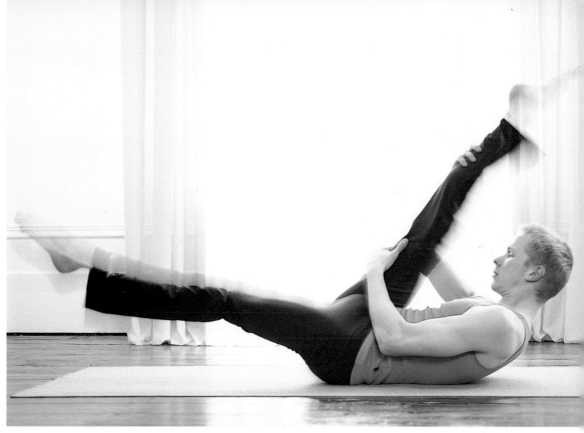

listening to your body

Practising different parts of the programme on a daily basis throughout your life will help you achieve a balance between strength and flexibility. As you practise the exercises and stretches, your awareness of your body, your movement style, your limitations and your qualities will become clearer and can make you your most experienced teacher – you will know what is best for you at any given time. You will have a body that is intelligent, responsive and intuitive.

The body does not lie. If something is not comfortable, if there is pain or excessive effort, it is not the right moment for a particular exercise or stretch. Forcing something will only lead to injury or overuse of a part of the body. This will then set up an undesirable pattern within the whole body, which will prevent it functioning at its best. Listen to your body; it has an amazing memory of all experience, including physical, intellectual, emotional and movement. Allow your body and mind to connect during exercise and you will develop an integration of both in all areas of your life.

how to use this book

The programme outlined in this book is structured so that you can focus on either developing strength or creating flexibility, depending on your needs. Alternatively, you can develop stability and suppleness of either the lumbar and pelvic region or the upper torso by following the specialized programmes at the end of the book. However you choose to train, you should first develop an innate knowledge of the fundamentals of the programme. It is also important to maintain your consistency throughout and progress in line with your body's responses, as this will prevent injury and inefficient patterns of movement. Aim to practise parts of the programme daily, and to do the whole programme when time permits.

The programme contains over 50 exercises and stretches, grouped into three main categories – fundamentals, developing strength, and creating flexibility – which focus on facilitating flexibility, strength and awareness of your body in both sustained postures and dynamic function to allow you to move with efficiency, grace and quality of movement.

fundamentals

The fundamentals are the basis for all the exercises. They teach you:

- how to align the spine and the skeletal structures
- how to release muscle work and tension
- the use of the breath in muscle work and developing rhythm
- how to develop patterns of muscle work
- and, most importantly, integration of the mind and body in movement.

It is essential to learn the fundamentals before you progress to the exercises, and to review them periodically even when you have achieved a high level of skill.

developing strength

The exercises in this section are derived from Pilates mat work, and help with the development and endurance of the transversus abdominus and lumbar multifidus muscles, which stabilize the spine and pelvic girdle in both static postures and dynamic movement. The exercises strengthen the abdominal and spinal muscles, creating a strong centre and a basis from which all movement can occur. By focusing on developing core stability, you are able to condition the body as a whole, with both quality and efficiency, and reduce the likelihood of degeneration of the skeletal system.

creating flexibility

Stretching and elongating the spine and limbs helps to develop body awareness, improves the alignment of the body and, in conjunction with strengthening, can correct muscle imbalances that may have developed through inappropriate use. Stretching also improves the range of motion within a joint and helps to prevent strained muscles. Flexibility depends on the relationship between your bones, connective tissue and surrounding muscles. It is dependent on many factors, such as posture, weight, age, degeneration, repetitive motion, lifestyle and previous injury, and is highly variable, not just among individuals. The flexibility of different joints within an individual can vary greatly, and also within the same joints on opposite sides of the body.

specialized programmes

lumbo-pelvic programme

This programme develops techniques from a wide range of disciplines to strengthen, stabilize and improve functional movement of the lumbar spine and pelvic region. Its aim is to prevent injury from repetitive overloading of the lower spine and to help recovery if there is a pre-existing injury.

shoulder girdle/upper torso programme

This programme includes various techniques to release, stabilize and protect the neck from overuse and misuse when working through the upper body, and also to strengthen the upper torso and improve its coordinated function.

When exercising, always remember:

- Joint capsules and ligaments may not return to their optimal length if they are overstretched, because of their elasticity; therefore the risk of injury is increased during exercise.

- Ideally, lengthening a muscle should be done gradually and should involve a slow sustained posture. Fast or bouncing movements may result in a shortening of the muscle, because of reflex responses.

- To release a muscle, the joint involved should not be taken to the end of its range of motion and it should be completely supported.

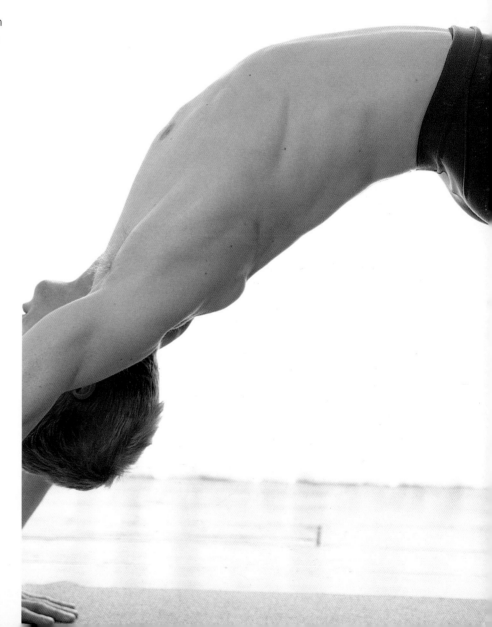

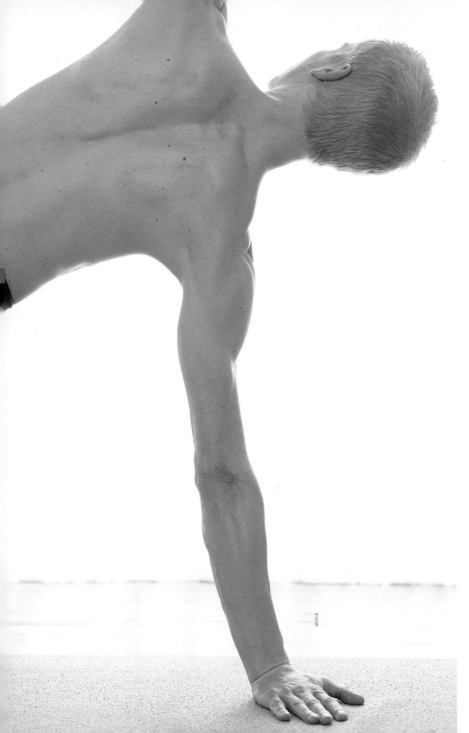

getting started

creating a comfortable environment

You will need an area where you can lie down with enough room to move freely without restriction. Lying on a mat or folded towel will help to support the body. You may also wish to support your neck with a towel or pillow, particularly if you have a history of neck pain or stiffness. The area you choose should be free of distractions, such as phone or television. The temperature of the room is also important – it is better to be too warm than too cold when exercising.

clothing

You should wear comfortable, loose-fitting clothing that doesn't restrict your movement. It is preferable to work with bare feet, as this will improve the sensory feedback of the feet in weight-bearing postures.

music

Some, though not all, people prefer to exercise to music. Music can help to develop a sense of rhythm and create a certain atmosphere, which may be to focus the mind and body or to create an integration of the body with music for more dynamic work. The choice of music is entirely your own – just be aware of its influence, as it can make all the difference to your focus and the outcome of your training.

breathing

The breathing pattern used in Pilates is known as thoracic or rib breathing, and is distinct from that used in other disciplines such as yoga. The aim is to keep your abdominal and spinal muscles engaged and your shoulders relaxed while your ribcage expands as you inhale. As you exhale the ribcage contracts down towards the waist, again involving the spinal muscles and also the pelvic floor muscles. The breathing also allows you to achieve a rhythm with the exercise. You do not need to practise this type of breathing at all times to the exclusion of all other breathing patterns – to be able to breathe in a variety of ways is more practical – but it forms an integral part of the Pilates exercises. If you have any respiratory conditions, such as asthma, it is better to breathe naturally than to impose a structured pattern of breathing.

fluids

It is important to drink plenty of water during and after exercise, particularly in hot climates. Still water is preferable to carbonated fluids.

nutrition

Nutrition affects your performance both physically and mentally. It is about providing your body with what it needs – no more, no less. You should try to avoid fatty foods, sugar and stimulants such as caffeine, and to minimize your intake of dairy and refined foods. A healthy diet is one that contains balanced amounts of protein, carbohydrates, fruits, vegetables and grains. Eat small amounts, and often, and eat foods that are organic (where possible), raw and unprocessed. The programme is not geared towards weight loss, although this may be a welcome by-product.

creating a routine

Structure the programme so that it fits in with the other activities in your life, for example first thing in the morning or after work. If you break your routine, try to get back into a pattern as soon as possible.

If you work long hours, and particularly if you are sitting for prolonged periods, try to get up and walk around every 30 minutes, or do a few gentle stretches for areas that are prone to tightness or pain, for example the lumbar spine or shoulders.

Develop a knowledge of how your body works during exercise, focus on specific muscles and movement patterns, and then begin to integrate your understanding into everyday activities. For example, you can correct your posture while sitting at your desk and lengthen your spine as you walk.

pain

Pain, and how it is perceived, is greatly influenced by attention, suggestion, previous experience, cognitive processing and anticipation – far more than any other sensation. Pain during exercise, however, is a possible indication that the body is at risk of damage or injury. You may be able to relieve symptoms if you exercise within a smaller range or use an alternative movement pattern, but if the pain is persistent, you should discuss it with your medical practitioner.

existing medical conditions

It is a good idea to consult your medical practitioner before starting any new exercise programme. You should always do this if you are receiving treatment for a medical condition, or if you are pregnant or taking any form of medication. Contraindications to exercise may include joint, muscle, bone, disc or back injury, high blood pressure, anaemia or other blood disorders, thyroid disease, diabetes, cardiac arrhythmia or palpitations, or epilepsy.

age and fitness

Your age and level of fitness are not an issue in the Pilates programme, as there are ways to modify the workout to fit your individual physicality and goals. Take responsibility for yourself as you exercise and do not force yourself beyond your limits – you know your body better than anyone else and, with practice, you can refine your knowledge of your strengths and limitations and progress appropriately. However, if you experience any discomfort or have difficulty with a particular movement or exercise, it is a good idea to consult your medical practitioner.

The following symptoms and signs are an indication that you should stop exercising and seek medical advice:

- pain
- faintness
- bleeding
- rapid pulse on resting
- dizziness

- back pain
- shortness of breath
- palpitations
- difficulty in walking

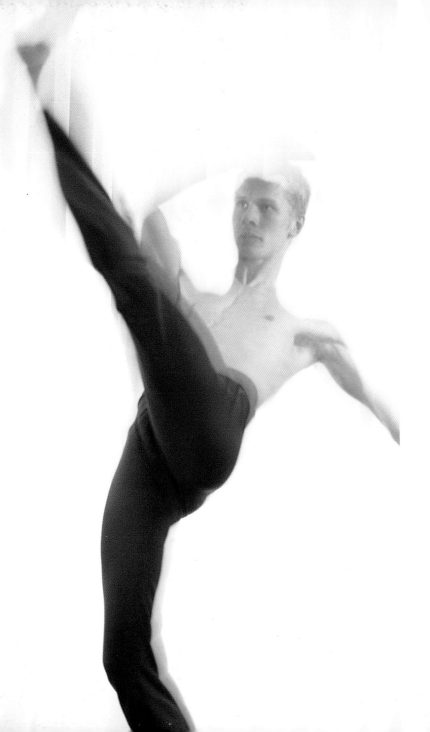

fundamentals

fundamentals

The fundamentals will help you to understand the principles of stability and efficient functional movement, and their integration into exercise and everyday activities. If you practise them every now and again you will develop a sense of the real essence of the Pilates-based programme for the spine. Read through each of the fundamentals described below, visualizing the movements, and then work through the exercise described in the second paragraph of each section.

alignment

Aligning the body will help you to gain an impression of where you may be holding tension in the muscles. It will also tell you whether you favour one side of your body in terms of strength or use of weight, the configuration of the spine, and will help you compare the symmetry of the same structures on the right- and left-hand sides of your body. It teaches you to be aware of your body before you start to exercise, so you have an internal knowledge of your strength, your sense of balance, and the relationship of your muscles to the joints they move.

Lie on the floor on your back with your arms by your sides, hands resting palms up, your legs hip distance apart and parallel, the neck lengthened with its natural curve maintained, your head in the midline, and your weight through your right and left sides equally. Sense the space beneath your lumbar spine and the height of the left and right pelvis. Allow the shoulders to release so that the shoulder blades are in contact with the floor; then release the chest and the jaw.

neutral pelvis

Neutral pelvis is an alignment of the pelvis which allows the lumbar spine to remain in an optimal position for function, which is neither flexed (pressing into the floor) nor extended (arched from the floor). This position reduces the amount of load through the spine and allows the abdominals and spinal muscles to work efficiently to support the spine, and balance the joints and surrounding muscles. You should try to attain this at all times with the exercises, unless you are working on a particular pattern of movement of the spine such as flexion – when you move out of flexion, attempt to return to neutral.

Focus on the space behind the lower spine, and imagine you can place your hand between your spine and the floor. Slide your hand under your spine, with the palm down. Your front pelvic bones should feel horizontal to the floor and at the same height on the left and right sides. Slide your hand out, maintaining the slight curve in your lumbar spine, and start to send your breath into this area to release and relax the muscles around the lumbar area.

transversus and multifidus co-contraction

The transversus working with the multifidus contributes to spinal stability and control of the segments of the lumbar spine. Studies have shown that the central nervous system controls these muscles. Integration of the functioning of these two muscles provides a basis for generating efficient movement and reducing the incidence of injury and skeletal degeneration.

Contract the abdominals in the area below the navel to the pubic bone, hollowing the muscle towards the spine so that the area below the navel flattens and widens. Sense the multifidus muscles working in conjunction with the

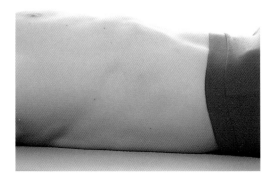
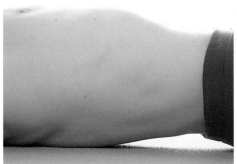

transversus muscle. Maintain both this contraction and the neutral pelvis alignment, and begin to incorporate the breathing pattern.

scapular stabilization

Stabilizing the scapula in its most functional position on the ribcage helps to maintain correct alignment of the shoulders and cervical spine. It also develops the involvement of the upper torso muscles (including the latissimus dorsi and serratus anterior) to reduce the effort of the smaller muscles (such as the trapezius) when working the upper body. Scapular stabilization plays a crucial role in posture, and it can help to prevent muscle fatigue during activities such as working at a computer, where repetitive movements cause overuse of the muscles and can lead to conditions such as repetitive strain disorder. In conjunction with stabilization of the pelvis, stabilizing the upper torso creates strength in the whole torso for challenging work, and prevents injury by balancing the upper and lower torso.

Lie on your back with the spine lengthened, the shoulders released, the neck long and the chest open. Raise your arms vertical to the shoulders and reach directly upwards so that the shoulder blades glide around the ribcage, then allow the shoulder blades to drop back to the floor, contracting the latissimus dorsi. Repeat the movement while contracting the abdominals, ensuring that you maintain a neutral pelvis and keep the ribs relaxed. Inhale as you reach up and exhale as you drop your shoulder blades back to the floor.

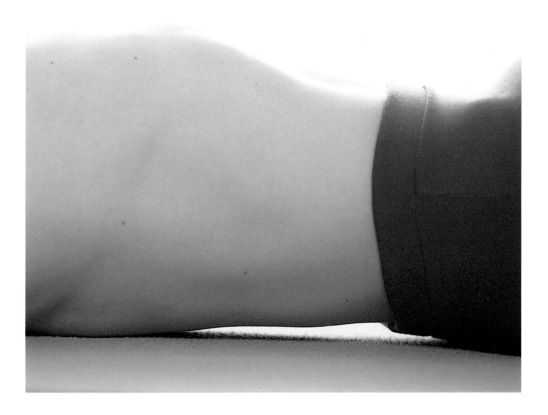

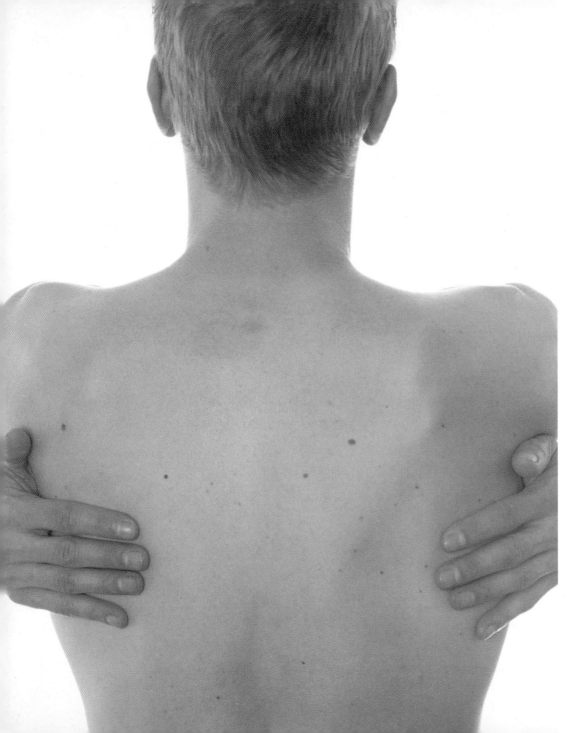

ribs and breathing

The ribs play a vital role in your ability to involve the abdominals accurately because of their relationship with the transversus muscle – the muscle attached to the lower ribs. The ribs also affect the alignment of the vertebrae because of their attachment to the thoracic spine. It takes time to be able to release the posture of the ribs by the use of the breath and abdominals, because you are often changing a breathing pattern that has existed for many years, and also because breathing is predominantly an automatic and unconscious process.

Place your hands across the lower ribs below the chest and be aware of their position and height. Begin to breathe in through the nose and exhale through a slightly open mouth. Continue to be aware of the ribs and their action during breathing. Now move your hands sideways to the sides of your ribs and as you inhale, feel the breath expanding into the sides, then exhale allowing the front of the ribs to release down to the pubic bone. Practise this pattern, and when you begin to get a sense of breathing sideways and releasing downwards on exhalation, practise breathing into the back of the ribs so that you can feel the ribs pressing into the floor.

You can practise this pattern intermittently throughout the day, when sitting or standing, but you should not aim to breathe like this all the time.

releasing the neck

Tension in the neck muscles and the associated jaw muscles can cause overuse or misuse of the cervical spine and its muscles. This can be a particular problem

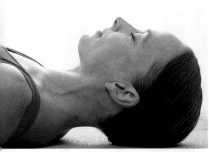

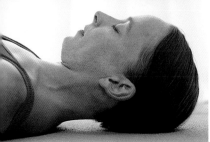

as the exercises become more challenging and involve working with the head lifted and therefore without support for the neck. Lengthening the neck and keeping a sense of its optimal alignment with the other vertebrae will help you to avoid overactivity of the small muscles of the neck and the upper shoulders. As you develop torso strength and control, it is common to compensate by tensing the shoulders, neck and jaw. As your strength and awareness develop, it will become easier to protect your neck. Progress slowly if you have any pain or stiffness after doing the exercises.

Allow your head to slide back along the floor, lengthening the front of the neck. Gradually flex the neck so that the chin moves to the chest and the back of the neck lengthens and releases.

working in turnout

Slightly turning outwards from the hip joint allows you to disengage the quadriceps muscle at the front of the thigh. This position strengthens the upper thigh, including the hamstrings, buttocks and rotators of the hip. It is an alternative position to working with the hips in parallel to isolate specific muscles. If you work in only one position, the body starts to establish habitual patterns of movement, so it is preferable to work in a variety of postures.

Turn your thighs outwards away from each other, with your feet in a small V-shape, heels together and knees released, and lengthen the legs. You should have a sense of working the entire torso.

pelvic floor

The pelvic floor is formed from internal muscles called the coccygeus and levator ani, which are attached to the pubic bone, the sacrum and coccyx, deep within the pelvic cavity. You need to exercise the pelvic floor regularly to maintain normal tone of the muscles. Pelvic floor exercises can be done in almost any position, including sitting, standing or lying down. Tighten the ring of muscle around the back passage and – in women – the ring of muscle around the entrance to the vagina. Pull up inside (imagine stopping the flow of urine), hold for five seconds, then release.

When exercising the pelvic floor, avoid holding your breath; instead, take a slow, deep breath in while contracting the pelvic floor, breathe out, and then release the muscles. Do not over-contract the abdominal and buttock muscles while contracting the pelvic floor. And avoid holding the pelvic floor muscles for more than five seconds, as they are fast-twitch fibres, which means they work optimally for short periods. Also avoid squeezing the legs together and tensing the inner thighs, as these are not directly attached to the pelvic floor.

fundamental
exercises

These fundamental exercises are the basis for the
Pilates programme and are designed to teach you
how to align the spine correctly, release tension,
develop patterns of muscle work, breathe in the
right way, and integrate your mind and body in your
movements. Come back to these exercises from
time to time, even when you have progressed to
the other exercises in the programme.

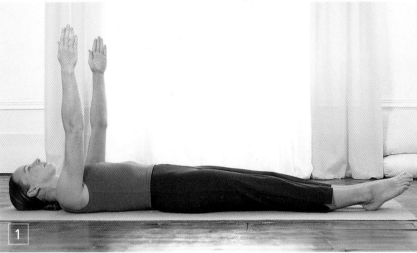

Step 1

Lie face up, legs extended and hip-distance apart. Contract abdominals and maintain pelvis in neutral, shoulder blades imprinting into floor, chest open. Raise arms to vertical.

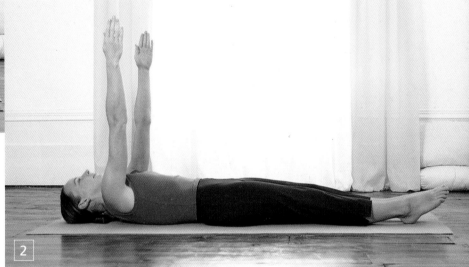

Step 2

Inhale, lengthen arms towards ceiling and then overhead, maintaining anterior ribs downwards and release of spine. **Exhale** to return arms to start position, contracting abdominals throughout and imprinting shoulder blades into floor.

arm lift to develop shoulder girdle stability, freedom of the shoulder joints and a sense of opening the chest

fundamentals

Step 1

Lie face up, palms facing hips. Draw shoulder blades down ribs, elongate spine, contract abdominals. **Inhale** to lift arms upwards in a circular shape, ribs released and spine lengthened.

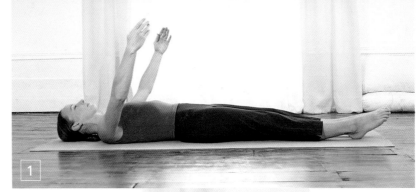

Step 2

Bring arms over head, maintaining circular shape.

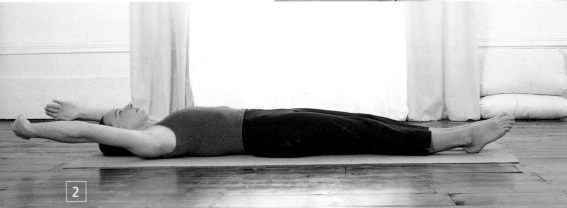

Step 3

Rest arms on floor behind head. **Exhale** to return arms to start position, keeping circular shape.

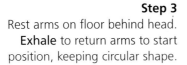

fundamentals

floating arms to open the chest and stabilize the shoulder girdle

48

Step 1
Lie face up, legs flexed and parallel. **Inhale**, draw shoulder blades down ribs, elongate spine, contract abdominals.

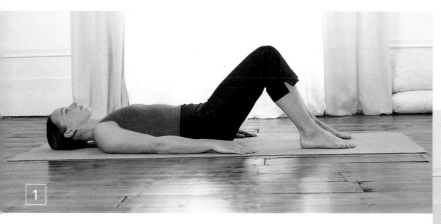

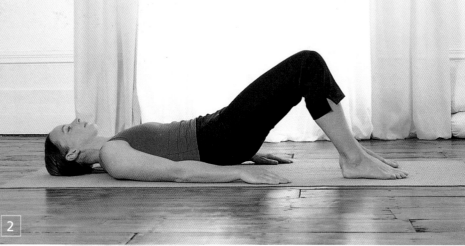

Step 2
Exhale to lift pelvis to level of waist, contracting abdominals, pelvic floor and hamstrings, pressing into whole foot.

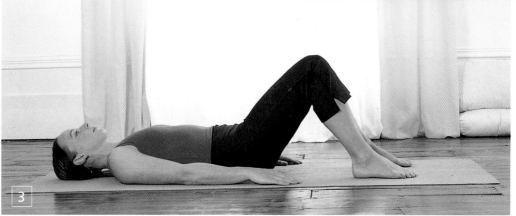

Step 3
Return to start position as you **inhale**.

Variation
Roll up, with the arms extended on the floor above the head. Alternatively, roll the spine up one vertebra at a time, starting at the base of the spine, and roll down in the same way to facilitate segmental mobility of the spine.

pelvic tilt to improve mobility of the lumbar spine and spinal stability

fundamentals

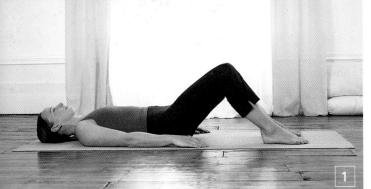

Step 1
Lie face up, legs flexed and hip-distance apart. Contract abdominals and maintain pelvis in neutral, shoulder blades imprinting into floor, chest open.

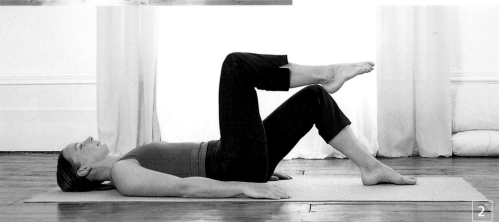

Step 2
Inhale, lift right knee towards chest until knee is in line with hip joint, maintaining neutral pelvis and release of spine.
Exhale to return leg to start position, contracting abdominals throughout and imprinting shoulder blades into floor.

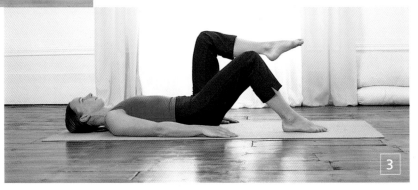

Step 3
Repeat on other side.

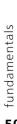

fundamentals

knee lift to develop a sense of neutral pelvis and spinal stability

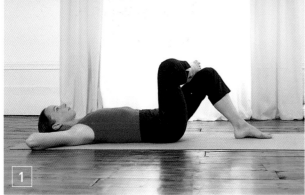

Step 1
Lie face up, left knee flexed, right ankle resting on left knee, pelvis aligned.
Open left hip as you elongate spine.
Place hands under head with elbows in direct contact with floor.

Step 2
Inhale to rotate legs to right, maintaining shoulder blade contact with floor, sensing rotation at waist, allowing pelvis to rotate freely.

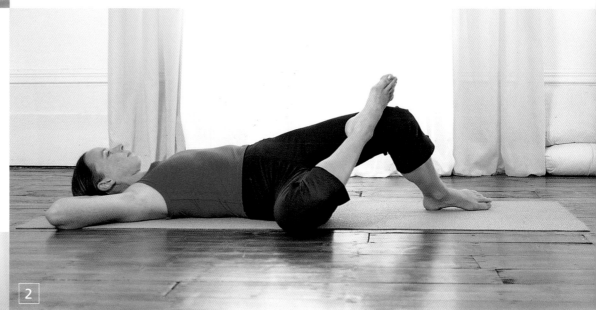

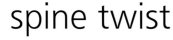

Step 3
Exhale to return to start position, focusing on drawing legs back, working left obliques to create the action.
After completing repetitions, repeat on other side.

spine twist

to strengthen the oblique muscles, to dissociate movement of the ribs and pelvis and to improve lumbar mobility

fundamentals

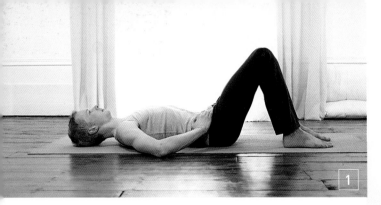

Step 1
Lie face up, both knees flexed.

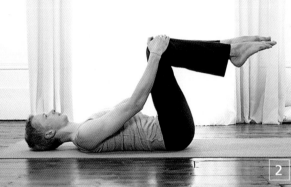

Step 2
Place hands on knees, draw knees towards chest, draw shoulder blades down ribs, elongate spine, contract abdominals.

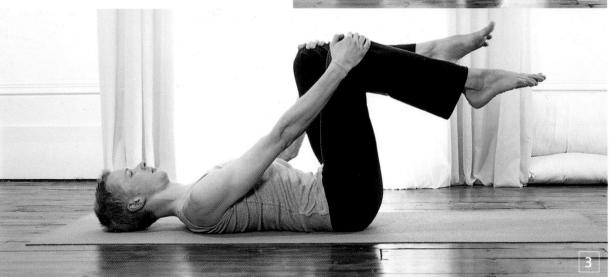

Step 3
Begin to push right leg away, resisting with right arm so there is minimal movement of leg, contracting upper hamstrings and buttocks as you push, **inhaling** and **exhaling** for 10 breaths maintaining contraction. Repeat on other side.

pelvic isometric
to improve stability of the lumbo-pelvic region and to develop symmetry of the pelvis and sacro-iliac joints

fundamentals

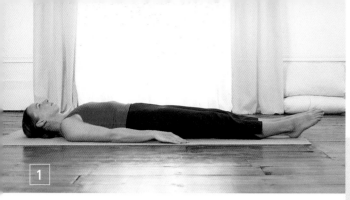

Step 1
Lie face up, legs hip-distance apart.
Contract abdominals and maintain pelvis in neutral,
imprinting shoulder blades into floor, chest open.

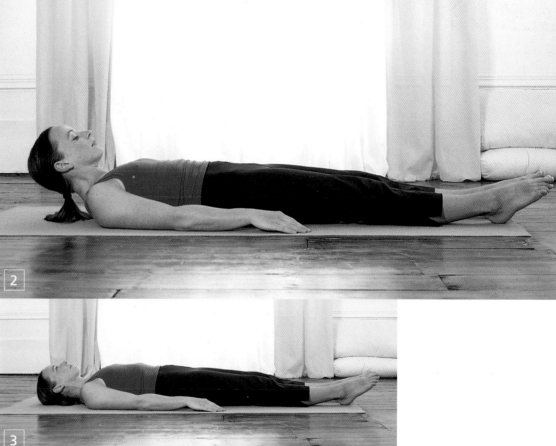

Step 2
Lengthen back of neck and
slightly draw chin towards chest.
Inhale to float head upwards
and slightly forwards, working
abdominals to achieve lift,
and release breastbone.

Step 3
Exhale to return to start
position maintaining support
for head via abdominals.

cervical curl to develop a sense of lengthening the neck and mobility of the cervical spine

fundamentals

Step 1
Lie face up, legs hip-distance apart, knees flexed, arms on floor, palms down. **Inhale**.

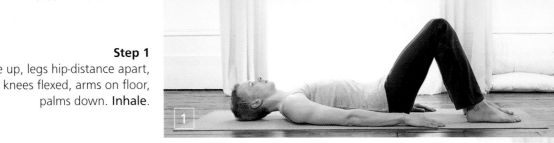

Step 2
Lengthen back of neck, contract abdominals, place hands behind head.

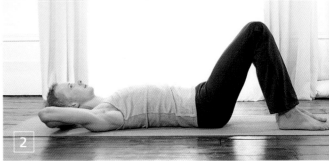

Step 3
Exhale and, supporting head with hands, raise upper body to tip of shoulder blades.

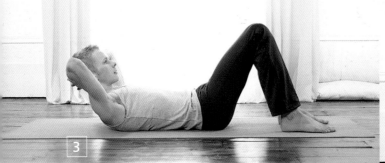

Step 4
Release anterior ribs and sternum towards pelvis, extend legs. **Inhale** to hold position, maintaining neutral pelvis and length of spine and neck. Return to start position as you **exhale** contracting the abdominals.

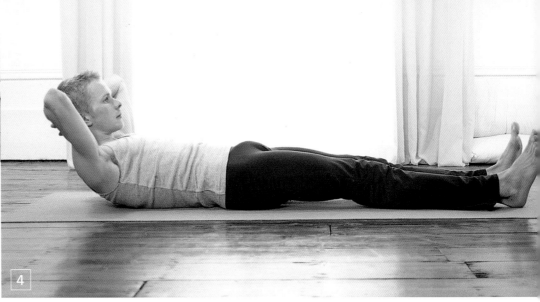

abdominal curl to facilitate strength of the deep transversus and rectus abdominis

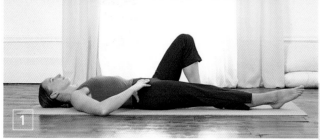

Step 1

Lie face up, legs hip-distance apart, left knee flexed. Contract abdominals and maintain pelvis in neutral, shoulder blades imprinting into floor, chest open.

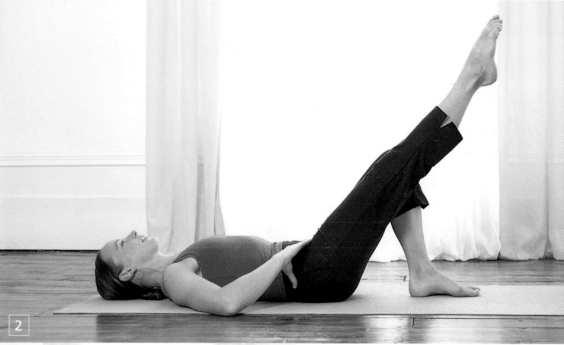

Step 2

Inhale, lift right leg to 45-degree angle to pelvis, maintaining neutral pelvis and release of spine.

Step 3

Exhale to return right leg to start position, contracting abdominals throughout and imprinting shoulder blades into floor. Repeat on other side.

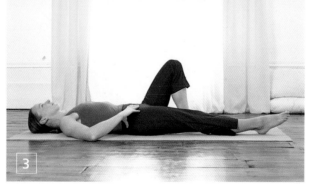

leg extension to develop a sense of neutral pelvis and co-contraction of transversus and multifidus

fundamentals

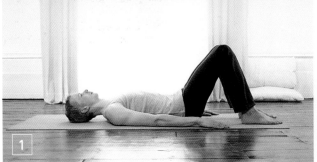

Step 1
Lie face up, legs flexed and parallel,
arms by sides, palms down.
Inhale, draw shoulder blades down ribs,
elongate spine, contract abdominals.

Step 2
Exhale to lift pelvis to level of
mid-spine, contracting abdominals,
buttocks and hamstrings,
pressing into whole foot.

Variation
Roll up with the arms extended on
the floor above the head
throughout the whole movement
(see right). Roll the spine up one
vertebra at a time and roll down in
the same way to facilitate
segmental mobility of the spine
(see far right).

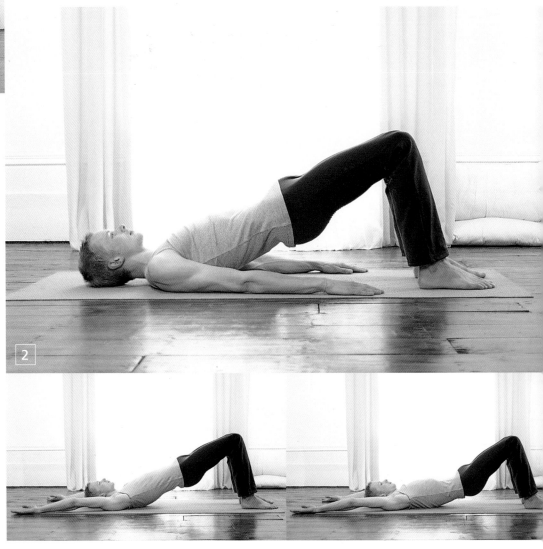

bridge to improve mobility of the lumbar spine and to strengthen the buttocks and hamstrings

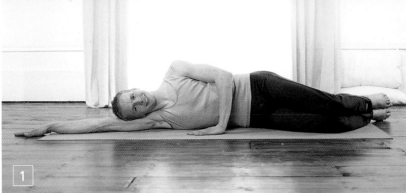

Step 1
Lie on right side, knees flexed and resting on top of each other. Contract abdominals, maintain pelvis in neutral, with shoulder blades released, right arm supporting head, left palm resting in front of chest. **Inhale**.

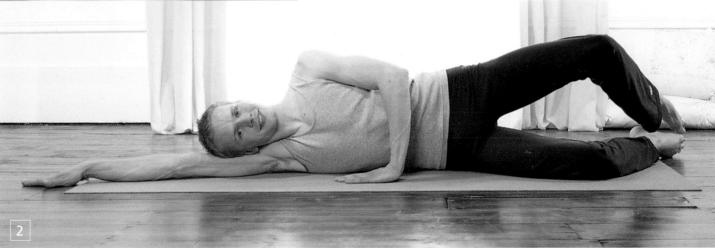

Step 2
Exhale to lift upper (left) leg, keeping ankles together and maintaining alignment of pelvis, contracting outer thigh and gluteals.

Step 3
Inhale to return to start position, maintaining contraction of legs and gluteals. Repeat on other side.

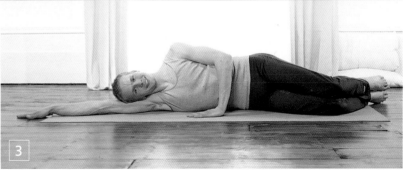

clam to develop lumbo-pelvic control and strength of the legs and gluteals

fundamentals

Step 1
Lie face down, with both palms resting near shoulders. **Inhale** as you draw shoulder blades down ribs, elongate spine, contract abdominals.

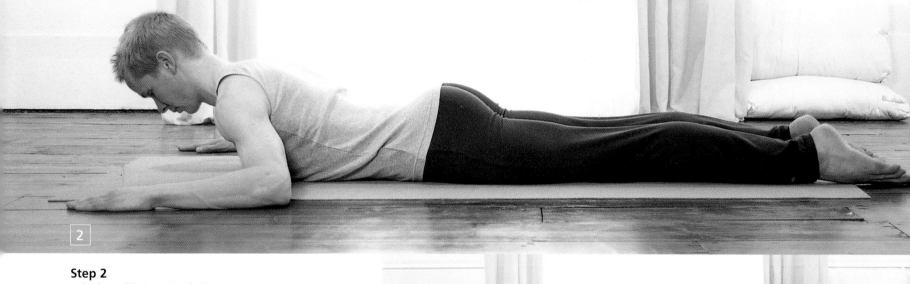

Step 2
Exhale to lift head and chest upwards as if extending sternum and allowing mid-spine to release, lengthen spine. **Inhale**.

Step 3
Return to start position as you **exhale**.

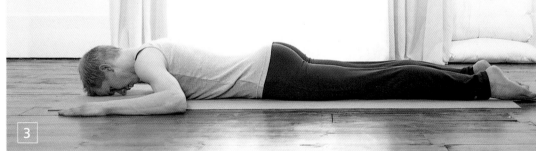

fundamentals

cobra to improve mobility of the mid-thoracic spine while opening the chest and stabilizing the shoulder girdle

Step 1
Lie face down, limbs extended,
arms by your sides, palms up.

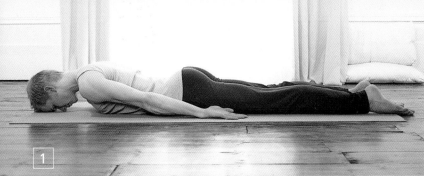

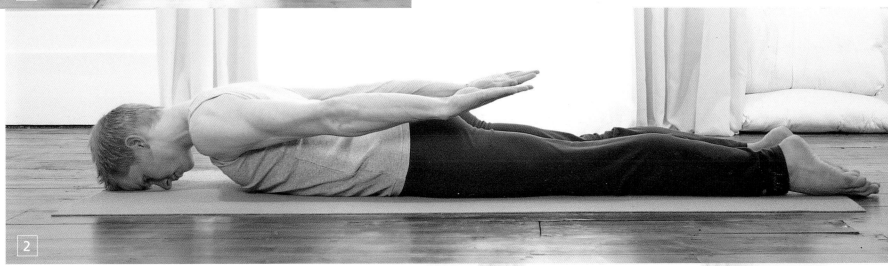

Step 2
Inhale, lengthen arms to hip height,
draw shoulder blades down ribs,
elongate spine, contract abdominals.

Step 3
Exhale to raise head
and chest from floor.
Lengthen arms towards feet
and maintain their height.
Inhale. Return to start
position as you exhale.

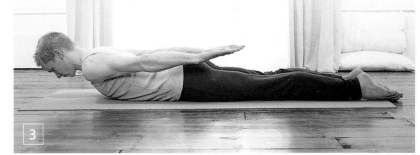

spine extension

to strengthen the spine extensors and to develop a sense of lengthening the lumbar spine when challenged in extension

fundamentals

Step 1
Sit with spine slightly flexed, arms extended at shoulder height, shoulders released, abdominals contracted, legs flexed at 45 degrees. Inhale.

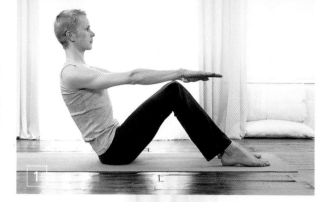

Step 2
Exhale, roll backwards onto pelvis and lower spine, contracting abdominals and maintaining release of shoulders. Inhale to hold position, increase abdominal contraction.

Step 3
Exhale to return to start position, contracting abdominals throughout and maintaining curve of spine.

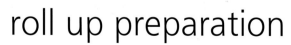

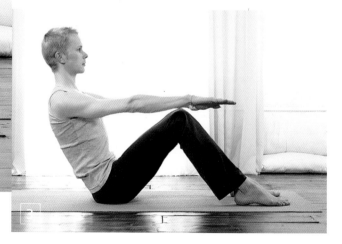

roll up preparation

to prepare for the roll up exercise (see p.76), to strengthen the deep abdominals and to improve awareness of the spine

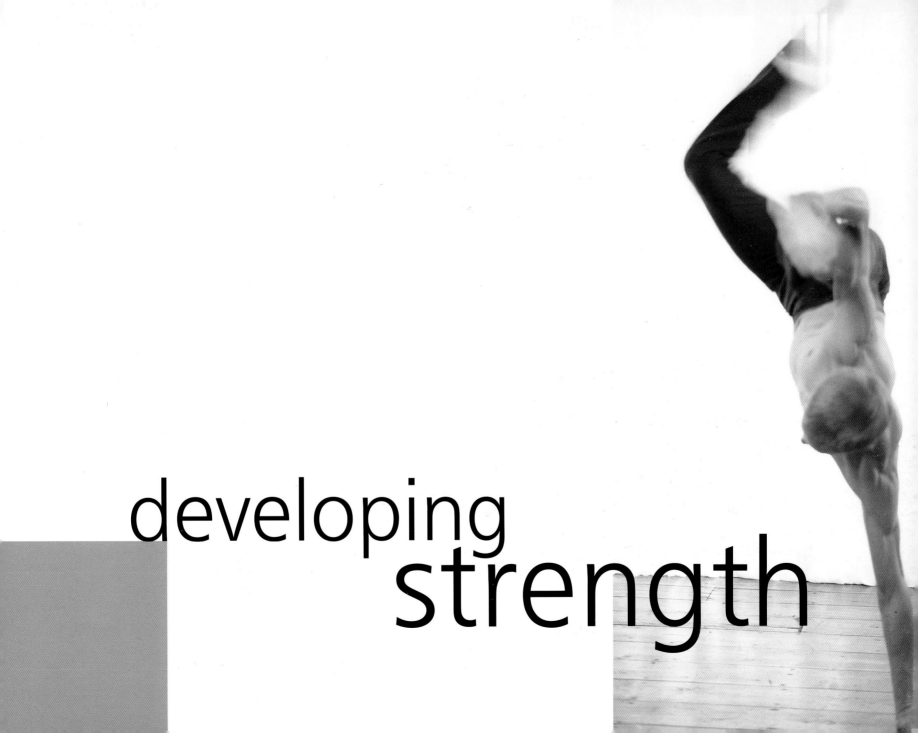

developing
strength

Step 1
Lie face up, legs extended, pelvis neutral.
Lengthen right leg to ceiling directly above hip
joint, releasing back of knee and maintaining
neutral pelvis.

Step 2
Inhale to circle leg inwards.

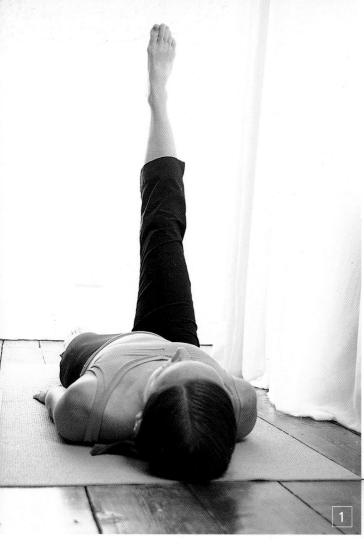

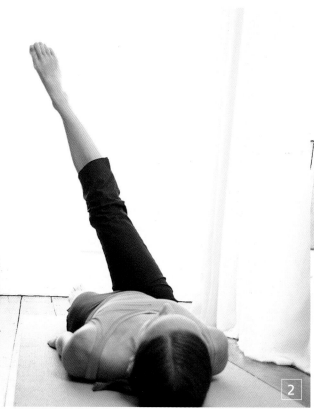

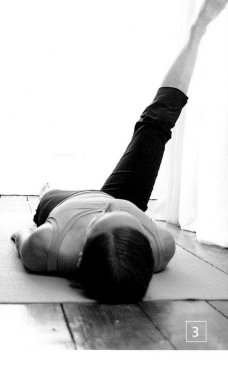

Step 3
Circle leg outwards to return to
start position, completing the
circle on **exhalation.**
Repeat, circling the leg outwards.
Repeat on other side.

single leg circle

to develop stability of the lumbar spine and pelvis, to improve motion of the hip joint and to strengthen the anterior leg muscle

Step 1

Lie face up, knees flexed and hip-distance apart. Contract abdominals, **inhale** to lengthen neck.

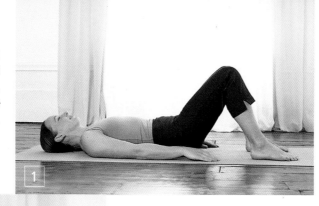

Step 2

Exhale, elevate head and chest, raise both legs, with right hand on outside of right leg and left hand on inside of right knee.

Step 3

Inhale to draw right leg towards chest. Extend left leg to 45 degrees, maintaining neutral pelvis. **Exhale** to change legs, transferring hands to other leg.

note

If you have a history of cervical injury or have current symptoms, leave the head supported on the floor.

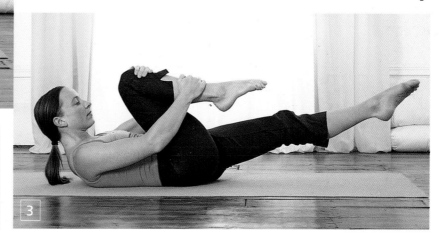

single leg stretch

to develop the strength of the deep abdominals and the rectus abdominis

developing strength
preliminary

63

Step 1
Sit with spine elongated, extend legs slightly wider than hip distance, feet flexed, arms extended at shoulder height. **Inhale**.

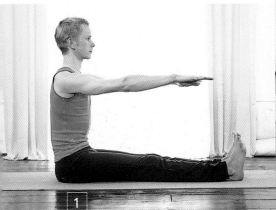

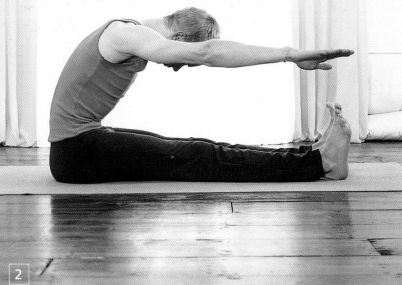

Step 2
Exhale. Flex the neck, continue flexing along length of spine from neck to sacrum, contract abdominals, lengthen arms.

Step 3
Inhale to reverse the movement, unfolding the spine.
Exhale to return to start position, lengthening limbs and spine.

note
If you have difficulty performing flexion it may be the result of tight hamstrings or reduced flexibility of the spine; improve the angle of the pelvis by sitting on a raised block until your mobility increases.

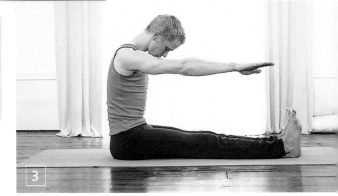

spine stretch forward

to facilitate spinal awareness and individual movement at each spinal segment while lengthening the hamstrings

Step 1
Lie on your right side, right arm extended on floor, left palm resting in front of chest. Lengthen spine and lower limbs, contract abdominals, draw shoulder blades down ribs.
Inhale.

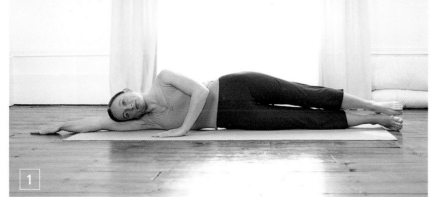

Step 2
Extend left leg upwards until in line with hip, contracting quads, slightly flexing foot.
Exhale to extend leg back to start position, maintaining neutral rib and pelvis position.
Repeat the exercise on the other side.

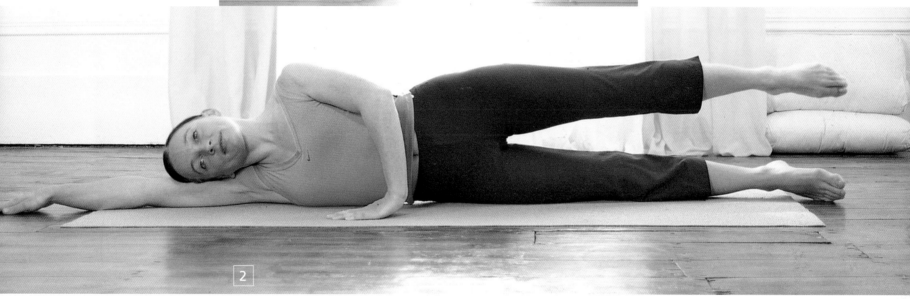

side leg lift to develop strength of the obliques and lumbo-pelvic stability unilaterally

developing strength
preliminary

65

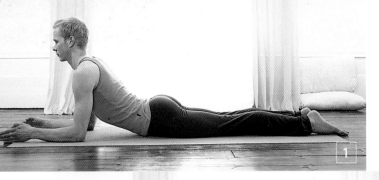

Step 1
Lie on your front with arms supporting upper body, contract abdominals, elongate spine and lift torso upwards. **Inhale**.

Step 2
Contract inner thighs and buttocks, raise right foot.

Step 3
Pulse right heel towards right buttock as you **exhale**, then lengthen right leg down to floor. Repeat with left leg. **Rest** in Spine Release Position (see p.102).

Progression
Perform the same movement with a double pulse, that is the heel moves in two beats towards the buttocks before returning to the mat.

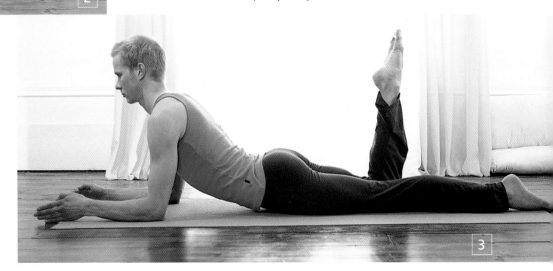

single leg kick

to develop strength of the hamstrings while facilitating spine extension and lengthening the hips and anterior torso

developing strength
preliminary

Step 1

Lie face up, knees flexed and hip-distance apart, contract abdominals. **Inhale** to lengthen neck. **Exhale**, draw knees in line with hip joints, extend legs upwards, feet pointed and crossed slightly, maintain neutral pelvis.

Step 2

Inhale to open the legs into a V lengthening from the hip joints, abdominals contracted. **Exhale** to return to the start position, tightening the inner thighs.

Variation

The movement can either be performed with the feet pointed or alternating between point and flex-point on opening, flexing at the ankle to return to the start.

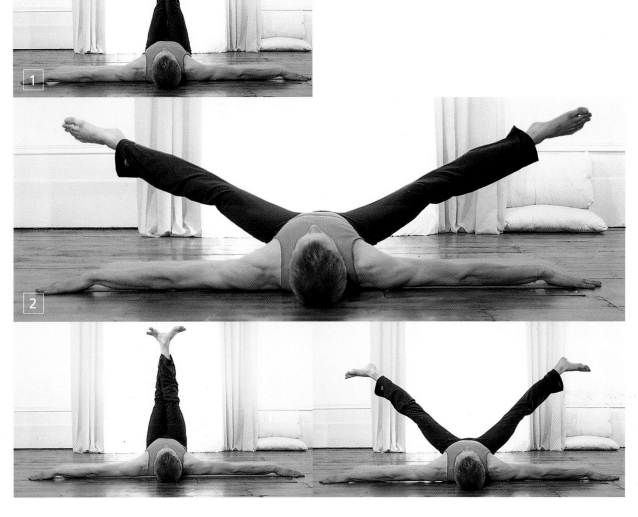

the V to develop the strength of the deep abdominals and the quadriceps

developing strength
intermediate

67

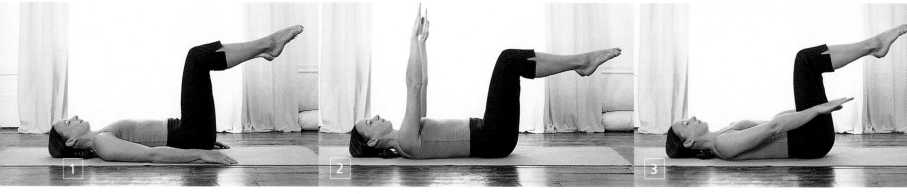

Step 1
Lie face up, pelvis in neutral, abdominals contracted, shoulder blades imprinting into floor, spine lengthened, legs elevated to 90-degree angle, knees directly in line with hips.

Step 2
Inhale, lengthen arms towards ceiling, imprinting shoulder blades into floor, contract abdominals, tighten buttocks and hamstrings, contract pelvic floor.

Step 3
Exhale, returning arms to start position, maintaining neutral pelvis.

note
If you have a history of cervical injury or have current symptoms, such as neck pain or stiffness, leave the head supported on the floor with Progressions 1 and 2.

Progression 1
Repeat with head and chest lifted as far as tips of shoulder blades, and legs extended above hip joints.

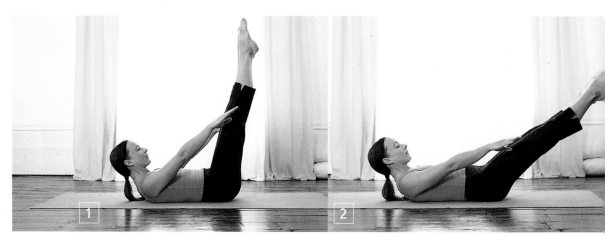

Progression 2
Repeat as for Progression 1 with legs lowered to a 45-degree angle to the hip joints.

developing strength
preliminary to advanced

the hundred
to strengthen the transversus and facilitate lumbo-pelvic stability

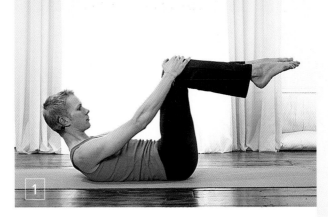

Step 1
Lie with knees directly above hip joints, head elevated, back of neck long, arms extended, hands placed below knees.

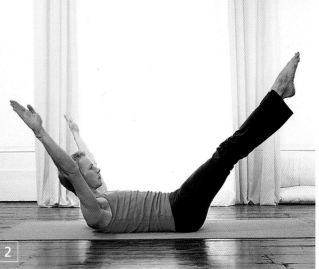

Step 2
Inhale to lengthen torso, extend arms wide overhead, lengthen legs to a 45-degree angle.

note

If you have a history of cervical injury or have current symptoms, support the head with a cushion or a rolled up towel throughout the exercise.

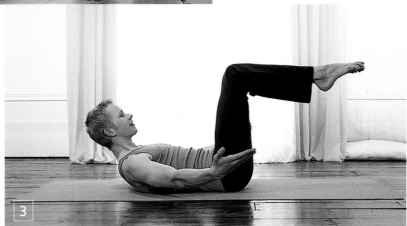

Step 3
Exhale, stabilize the pelvis, contracting the legs and buttocks, return knees to start position and circle the arms back towards knees.

double leg stretch
to strengthen and tone all layers of the abdominal muscle and develop coordination

developing strength
intermediate

69

Step 1
Sit with legs extended, spine lengthened, shoulders released, arms flexed in front, palms facing you.

Step 2
Inhale to roll backwards, maintaining a long curve in spine, contract abdominals, lengthen crown of head upwards.

Step 3
Maintaining shape of torso, first turn arms inwards, then extend them to sides.

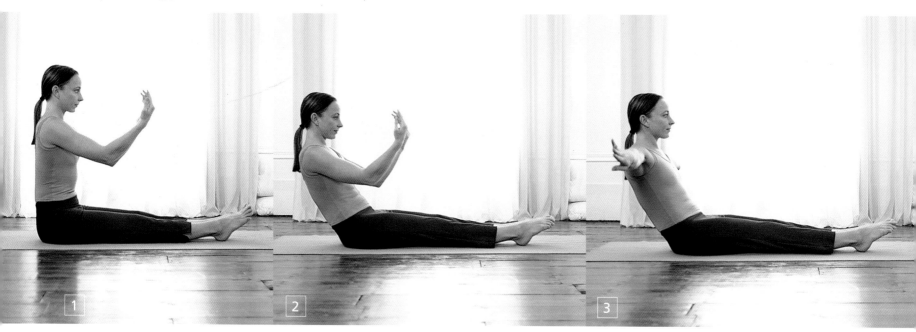

rowing

to develop the strength of the deep abdominals, to facilitate mobility of the spine and coordination of the torso and arms

Step 4
Exhale, stretch arms behind, palms up and extend the spine forwards.

Step 5
As spine flexes over legs, circle arms in a swimming motion towards feet. Roll back up to start position.

developing strength
intermediate

71

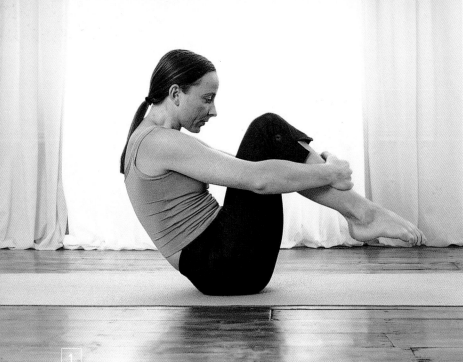

Step 1
Sit with knees flexed into chest, hands holding top of ankles with heels together, flex spine, contract abdominals, tuck chin to chest, maintain balance on sacrum.

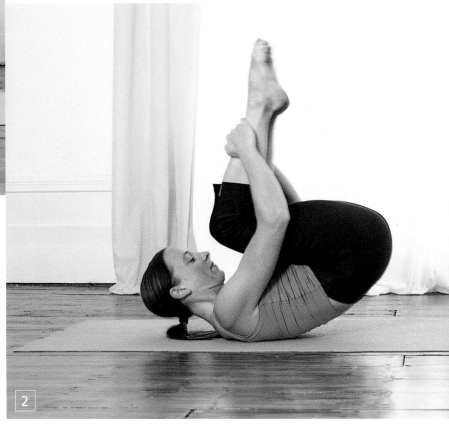

Step 2
Inhale to roll backwards to tip of scapula, remaining flexed through length of spine, knees slightly apart. Exhale to return to balance position, abdominals contracted, keeping flexed shape of body.

developing strength
intermediate

72

rolling like a ball to facilitate flexion of the spine and stabilization of the spine in dynamic movement

Step 1
Sit with knees flexed and shoulder-distance apart, holding ankles.

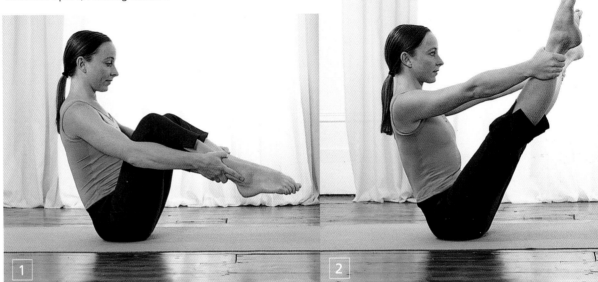

Step 2
Contract abdominals, lengthen legs upwards into V-shape.

Step 3
Inhale, flex neck, roll backwards along length of spine to tip of shoulder blades.
Exhale to return to Step 2, maintaining balance on base of sacrum before rolling back.

note

If you have a history of spinal injury or have current symptoms, such as pain or stiffness, limit the range of movement in the exercise until your strength and flexibility increase.

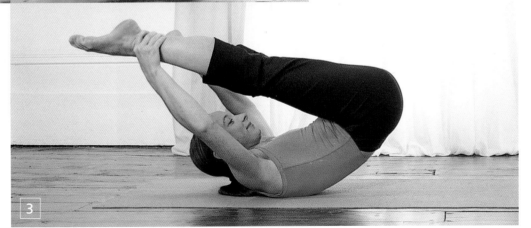

open leg rocker to mobilize and elongate the spine and facilitate strength of the transversus

developing strength
intermediate

73

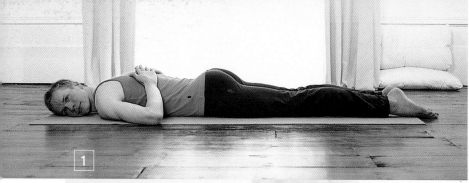

Step 1
Lie face down with head facing left, hands crossed over upper spine. Contract buttocks and inner thighs, drawing abdominals away from floor. **Inhale**.

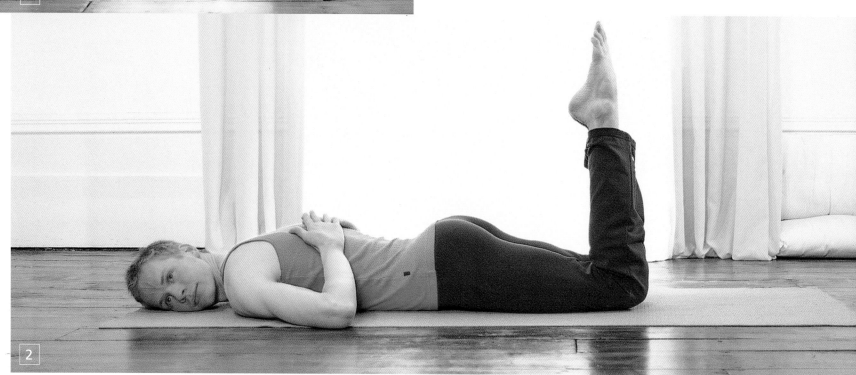

Step 2
Pulse heels towards buttocks for 3 beats, maintaining length through spine and contraction of abdominals.

double leg kick to strengthen the leg extensors and buttocks and elongate the spine

<table>
<tr><td>note</td><td>Extension movements of the spine may cause discomfort, so modify the exercise, for example by reducing range or number of repetitions. Avoid extension with spinal instability conditions.</td></tr>
</table>

Step 3

Exhale, extend legs back to floor, extend arms towards feet with clasped hands, arch upper body from floor.

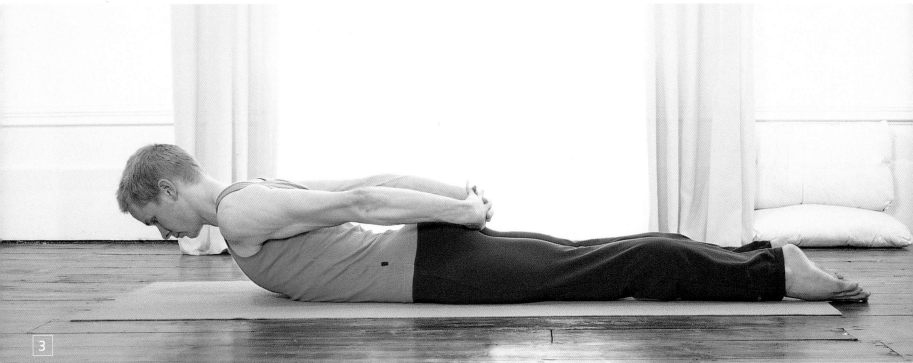

Step 4

Inhale to return to start position with face turned to right and repeat sequence, alternating turning of head. After completing repetitions **rest** in Spine Release Position (see p.102).

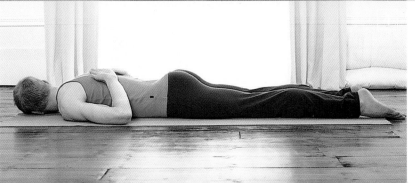

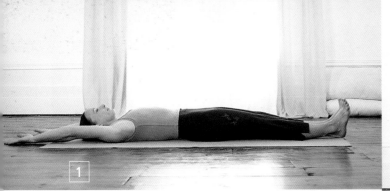

Step 1
Lie face up, legs and arms extended, pelvis neutral.

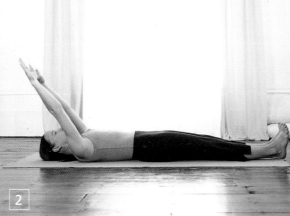

Step 2
Inhale, lengthen arms towards ceiling, elongate spine, contract abdominals, flex feet, tighten buttocks and inner thighs.

Step 3
Stretch arms forwards, curl neck, roll up and over legs. **Exhale** to lengthen spine lifting out of pelvis, shoulders released.

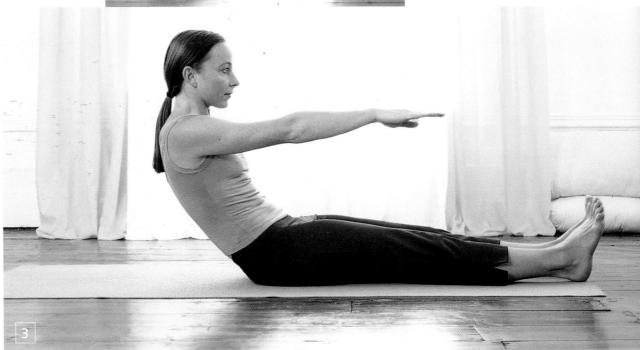

roll up

to develop a sense of dissociating movement of the torso from the pelvis and to facilitate shoulder girdle stability

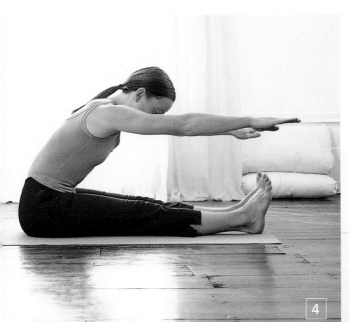

Step 4
Reach forward as far as possible.

Step 5
Inhale to reverse the movement, rolling back down one vertebra at a time, contracting abdominals, buttocks and thighs.

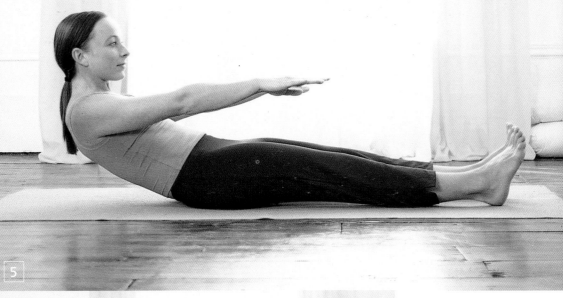

note

If you have a history of spinal injury, particularly involving the disc or neural structures, limit the forward movement, avoiding full flexion.

Step 6
Exhale to lower head to floor as arms return to start position, elongate limbs and spine.

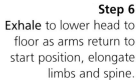
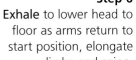

developing strength
advanced

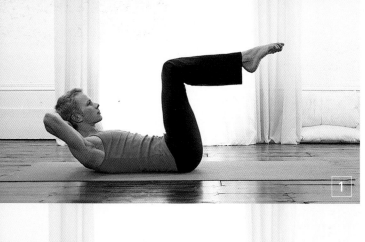

Step 1
Lie face up, knees flexed, legs hip-distance apart, abdominals contracted, pelvis in neutral, hands behind head. **Inhale**.
Exhale to raise head and upper spine, supporting head with hands, lift legs to 90-degree position, knees directly above hips.

Step 2
Inhale to rotate right scapula to left pelvis, extending right leg.
Exhale at end of movement.

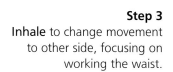

Step 3
Inhale to change movement to other side, focusing on working the waist.

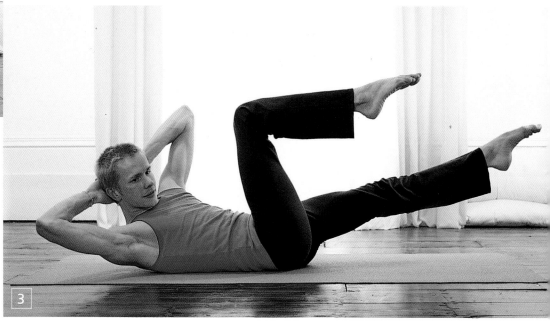

oblique twist

to develop strength of the obliques and to sculpt the abdominals and waist

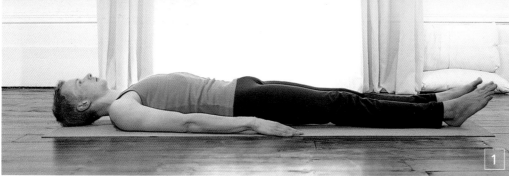

Step 1
Lie face up with legs and arms (palms down) extended, pelvis neutral, contracting deep abdominals. **Inhale**.

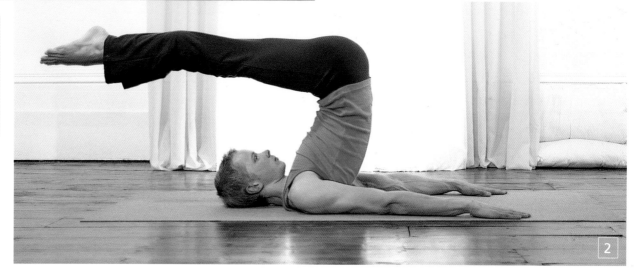

note

If you have a history of cervical injury, or are experiencing current symptoms, limit the range of the movement by rolling to middle of spine.

Step 2
Roll legs upwards and over head, extending legs in parallel, contract inner thighs and buttocks, maintaining weight through shoulder blades and pressing into back of arms for balance.
Exhale to open legs to hip-distance apart, roll back down one vertebra at a time, maintaining deep contraction of abdominals.
Lower legs to floor slowly, and return to start position.

Variation
Repeat the exercise with the legs in reverse: open the legs at hip distance to roll up and over head, closing the legs on the return to roll down.

roll over
to facilitate flexibility of the spinal muscles and mobility of the spine, balance and coordination

developing strength **advanced**

79

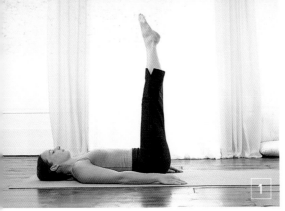

Step 1
Lie face up, legs extended, pelvis neutral.
Lengthen both legs to ceiling directly above hip joint, release back of knee and maintain neutral pelvis, contract buttocks and inner thighs.

Step 2
Inhale to begin circling legs to right.

Step 3
Circle legs right and down.

Step 4
Continue circle to left to return to start position, completing the circle on **exhalation**.

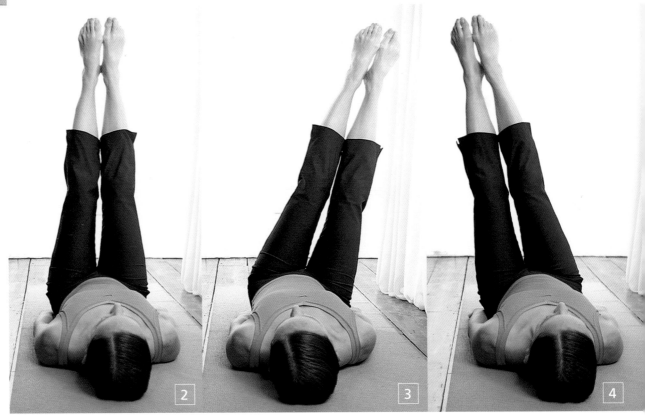

developing strength
advanced

80

corkscrew

to develop stability of the lumbar spine and pelvis, to improve motion of the hip joint and to strengthen the deep abdominals

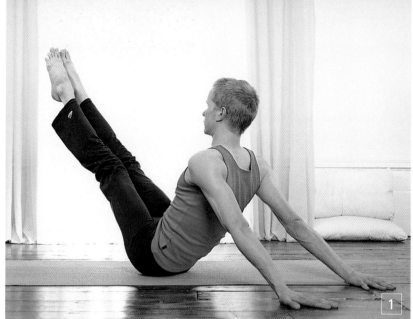

Step 1
Balance on sacrum with legs together at 45-degree angle to hips, extend arms behind trunk, pressing into palms.

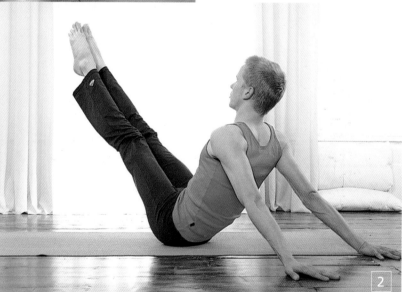

Step 2
Inhale to circle legs downwards and to right, maintaining arms in extension and length through spine. **Exhale** to continue circle round to left, returning to start position. Repeat circle starting to left. Alternate circles with each repetition.

hip twist to develop a deep strength of the abdominals and control of the lumbo-pelvic region

developing strength
advanced

81

Step 1

Lie face up, knees flexed and parallel.
Inhale, draw shoulder blades down ribs, elongate spine, contract abdominals.
Exhale to lift pelvis to level of mid-spine, contracting abdominals, buttocks and hamstrings, pressing into whole foot.

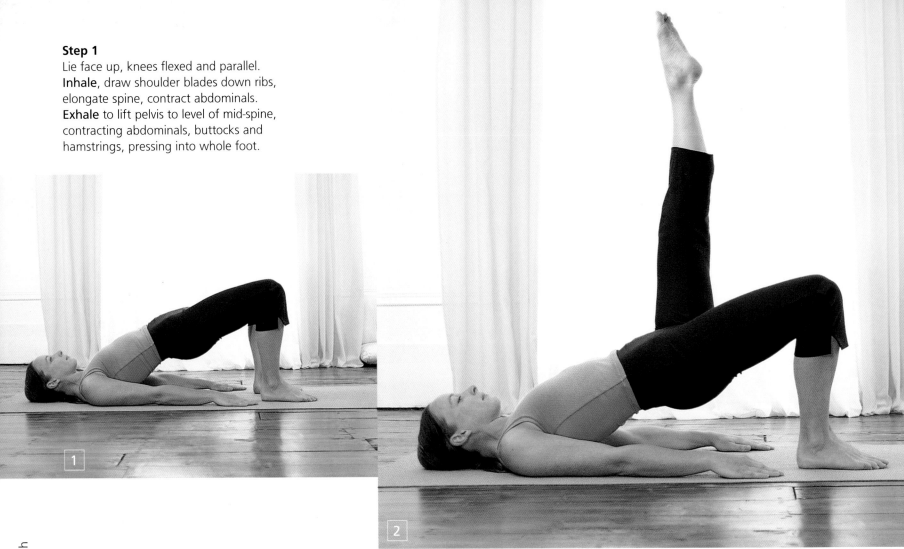

Step 2

Inhale to extend left leg upwards until vertical to mat.

shoulder bridge to improve mobility of the lumbar spine and to strengthen the buttocks and hamstrings

Step 3
Exhale and begin to lower left leg.

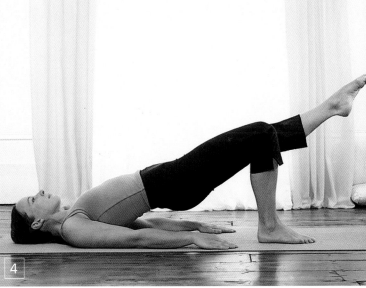

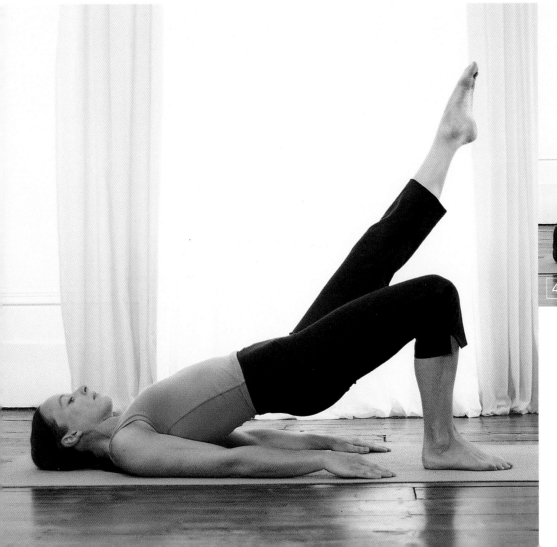

Step 4
Lower left leg until level with right knee.
Return to start position as you **inhale.**
Repeat on other side.

developing strength **advanced** 83

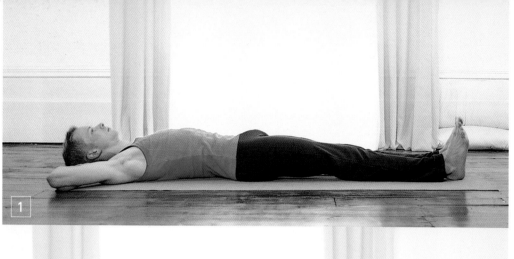

Step 1
Lie face up with hands supporting head, spine lengthened, legs hip-distance apart, feet flexed. Contract abdominals. **Inhale**.

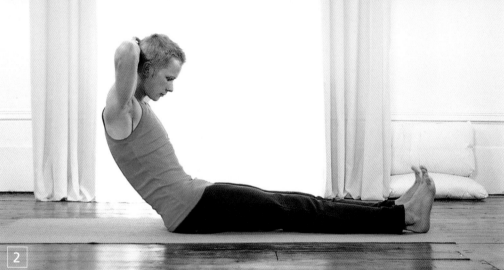

Step 2
Roll up, flexing spine from floor one vertebra at a time, contract buttocks.

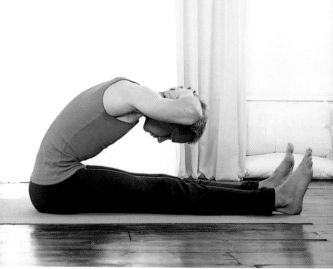

Step 3
Exhale to lengthen spine forwards over legs, keeping elbows wide.

neck pull to develop strength of the abdominals and facilitate spinal flexibility

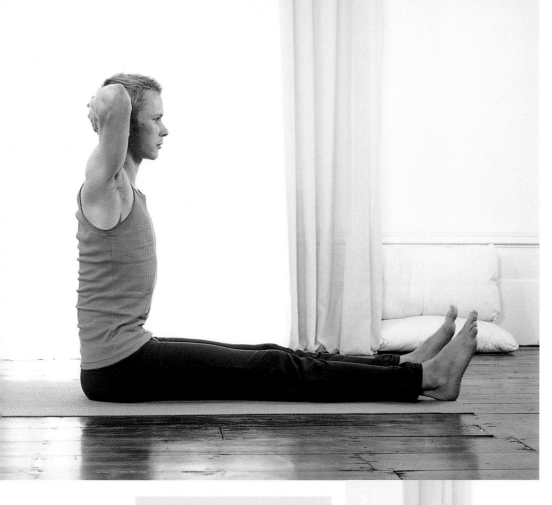

Step 4
Inhale to roll up to a lengthened position, reaching crown of head upwards.

Step 5
Exhale to roll down, one vertebra at a time to return to start position.

note
If you have current spinal symptoms or a pre-existing spinal condition, avoid full flexion during the forward movement, curling only half way, until your strength increases.

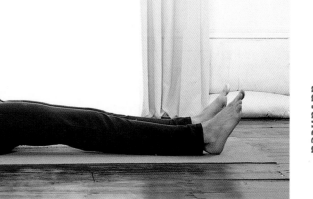

developing strength **advanced**

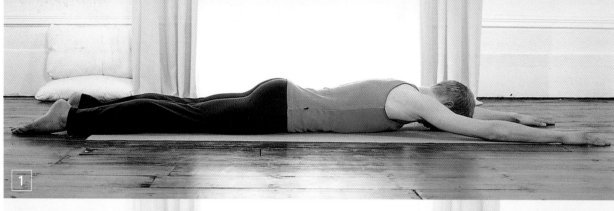

Step 1
Lie face down, arms extended over head, legs lengthened. Contract abdominals, elongate lumbar spine. **Inhale**.

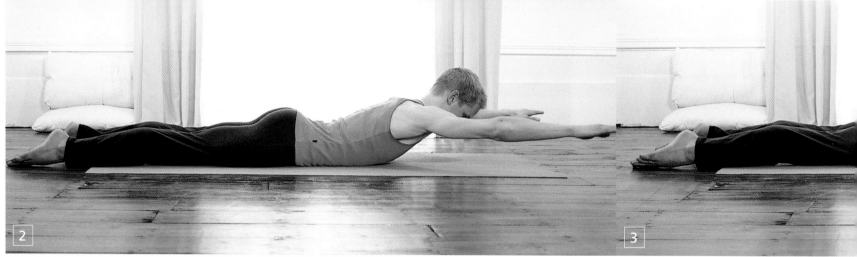

Step 2
Exhale to lift arms and upper body.

Step 3
Inhale to release neck, looking towards floor as arms circle towards hips.

breast stroke

to develop length and extension of the spine and to facilitate shoulder girdle stability

note If you have a discal condition, the extension movement of the spine may cause discomfort, so modify the exercise in terms of your range or repetitions. With instability conditions, avoid all extension movements.

Step 4
Exhale to flex elbows.

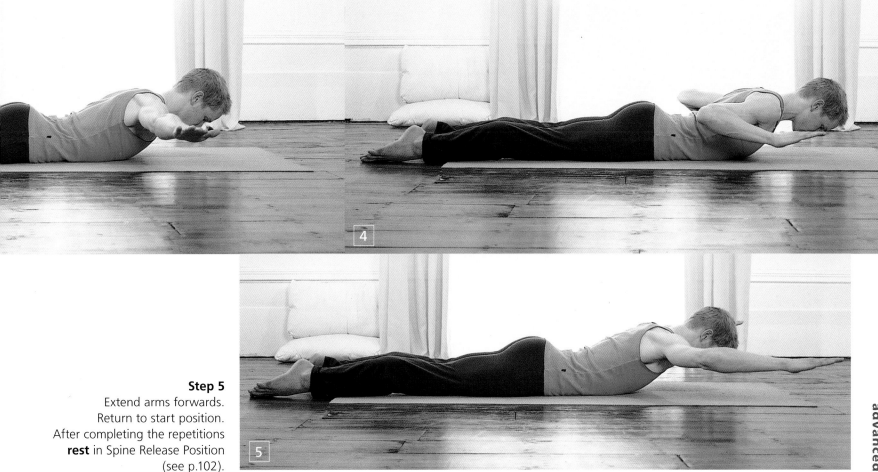

Step 5
Extend arms forwards.
Return to start position.
After completing the repetitions
rest in Spine Release Position
(see p.102).

developing strength
advanced

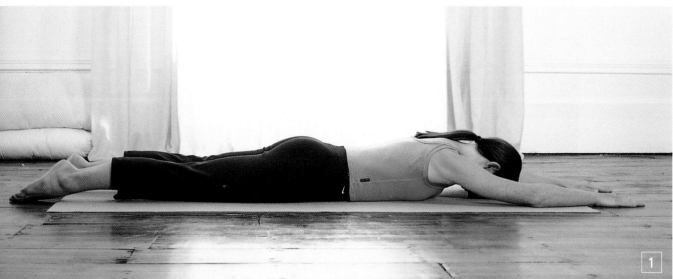

Step 1
Lie face down, legs lengthened. Draw shoulder blades down, extend arms forward, contract abdominals. **Inhale**.

Step 2
Exhale, lift left arm, right leg and head, keeping back of neck long, maintaining neutral pelvis as you lengthen limbs and elongate spine.

note

Swimming is a challenging exercise, utilizing the whole body in a very dynamic pattern, so develop the strength to perform the movements gradually. If you have a discal condition, the extension movement of the spine may cause discomfort, so modify the exercise in terms of your range or repetitions. Avoid extension with instability conditions such as spondylolisthesis.

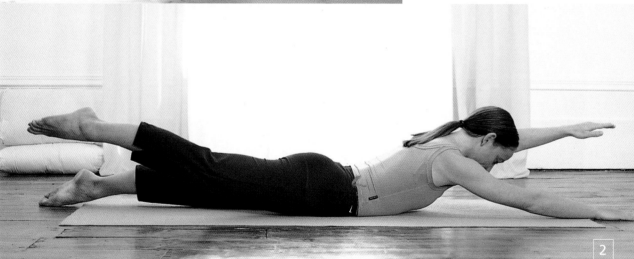

swimming to develop a sense of elongating the spine and to strengthen the spine extensors

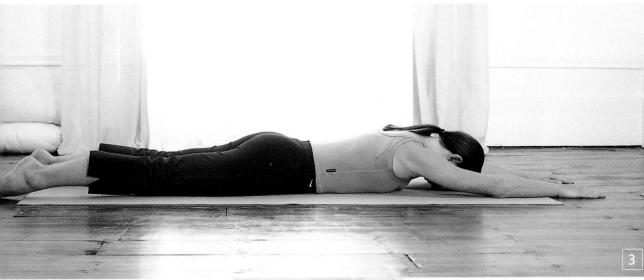

Step 3
Inhale to lower limbs and head to start position, maintaining length in spine and activation of abdominals.
Exhale to repeat on other side.

Progression 1
Lift all four limbs and head. Maintain position for 5 **inhalations** and 5 **exhalations** (see right).

Progression 2
Maintain position in Progression 1 and begin to alternate diagonal lifting of limbs, at double pace, without contacting mat; that is, perform an actual swimming motion. Continue motion for 10 **inhalations** and 10 **exhalations**.

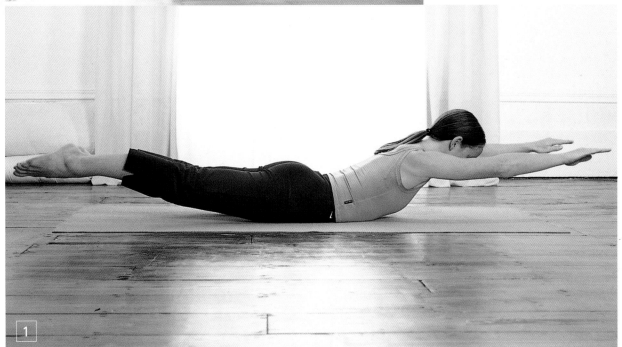

developing strength
advanced

89

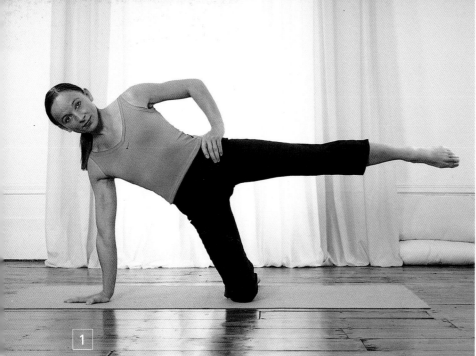

Step 1

Kneel on right knee, right palm resting on floor directly under shoulder, left hand resting on pelvis. Lengthen left leg in line with pelvis and ribs, contract abdominals. **Inhale**.

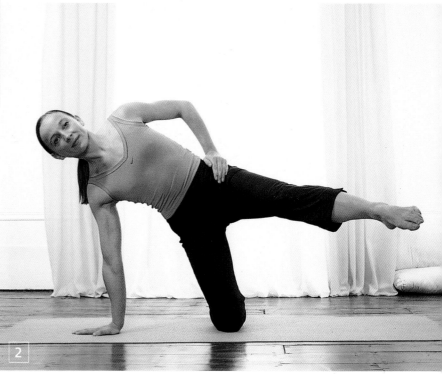

Step 2

Exhale to flex left leg forwards and then backwards with foot pointed, maintaining balance and alignment of torso. Repeat on other side.

note

If you have a knee condition, take care with kneeling positions and weight-bearing through the knees; kneel on a folded towel to give support to the joint.

developing strength
advanced

90

kneeling side kick to develop lateral strength of the trunk and hip muscles and to facilitate balance

Step 1
Sit with knees flexed to the side and left foot slightly in front of right foot. Place right palm on floor directly under shoulder. **Inhale**.

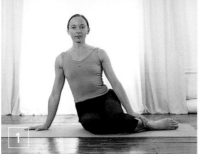

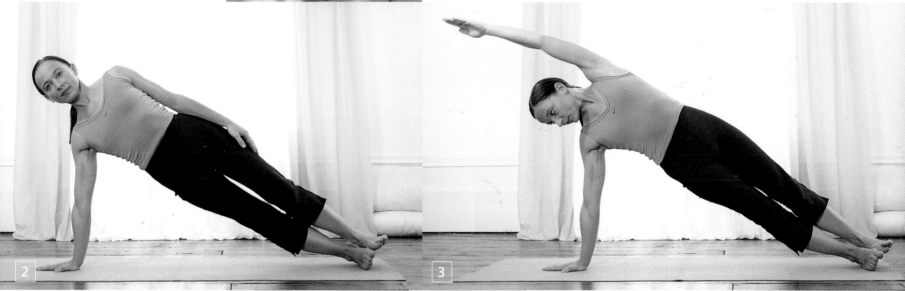

Step 2
Exhale to lift body, taking weight through right arm as it extends, extending legs and lengthening body from crown of head to feet. **Inhale**.

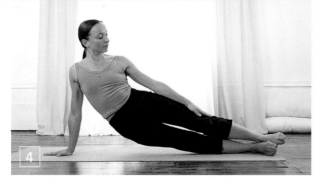

Step 3
Exhale to extend the left arm over head, lengthening arm and spine.

Step 4
Inhale to lower body to start position. Repeat on other side.

side bend to develop balance and strengthen the torso, obliques and upper limbs

developing strength **advanced**

91

Step 1
Kneel on all fours, palms directly below shoulders. Contract deep abdominals and extend legs until body is in a push-up position, weight through balls of feet.

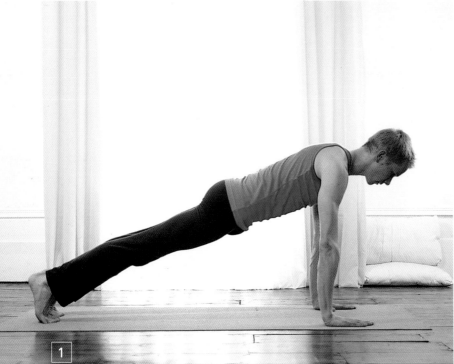

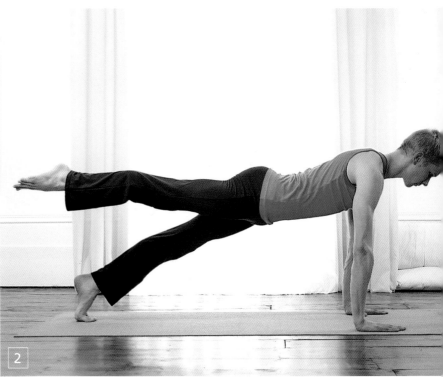

Step 2
Inhale to extend right leg upwards slightly higher than pelvis.
Exhale to return leg to floor Repeat exercise on left leg, returning to kneeling position to finish.

developing strength
advanced

leg pull down to develop strength in the arms and upper body, and in the spinal and leg extensors

Step 1
Sit with legs extended, spine lengthened, shoulders released, palms pressing into floor near pelvis. **Inhale** to lift pelvis upwards until legs and arms are fully extended, maintaining contraction of abdominals, buttocks and quadriceps.

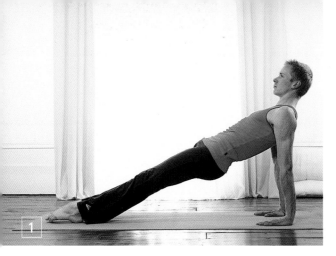

Step 2
Extend left leg upwards with foot pointed, maintaining level of pelvis so head and toe are at equal height. **Exhale** to lower left leg to just above floor and repeat movement.

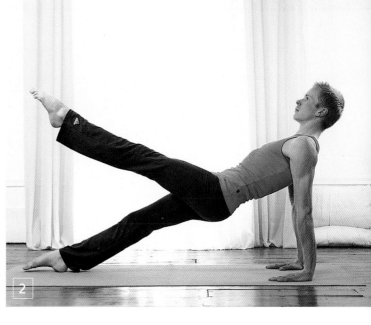

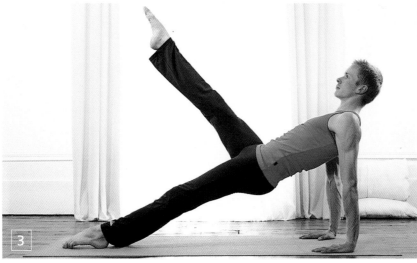

Step 3
Repeat on the right leg. Lower buttocks to floor to return to start position.

leg pull up
to develop power in the upper body, to facilitate pelvic control and quadriceps strength

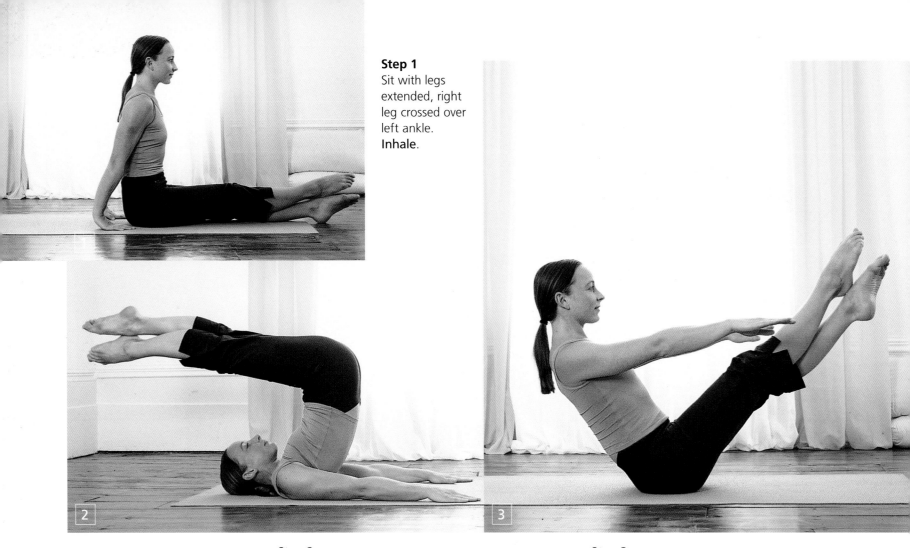

Step 1
Sit with legs extended, right leg crossed over left ankle. **Inhale**.

Step 2
Roll backwards, extending legs over head. **Exhale**.

Step 3
Inhale and roll up into V position, lengthening arms towards feet.

boomerang
to develop flexibility of the spine, strength of the torso and coordination of the body

Step 4
Balance, circle arms behind back, clasp hands.

Step 5
Exhale and lean forward, lowering legs to floor, stretching body over legs, stretching arms behind.

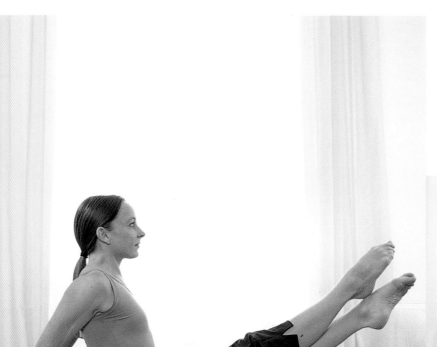

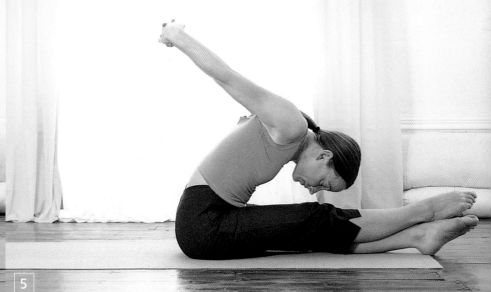

note If you have a history of spinal injury, or have current symptoms, limit the range of the exercise and minimize the repetitions until your strength and coordination develops.

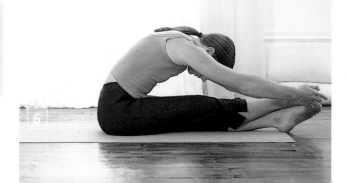

Step 6
Circle arms forwards, reaching to toes. Return to start position.

developing strength **advanced**

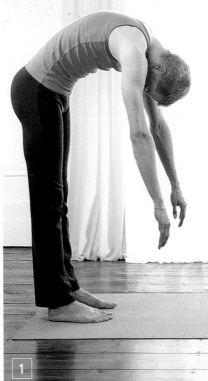

Step 1
Stand with feet hip-distance apart, contract abdominals. **Inhale**. **Exhale** to flex forwards.

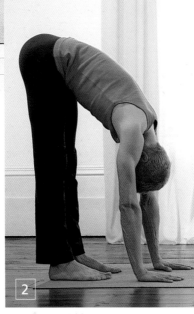

Step 2
Place palms on floor in front of feet.

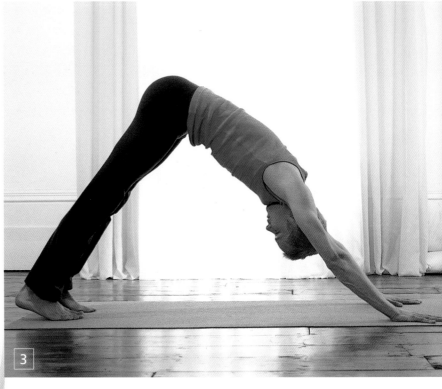

Step 3
Inhale to walk hands forwards.

push up to improve strength of the upper limbs, chest and upper back and facilitate flexibility of the hamstrings

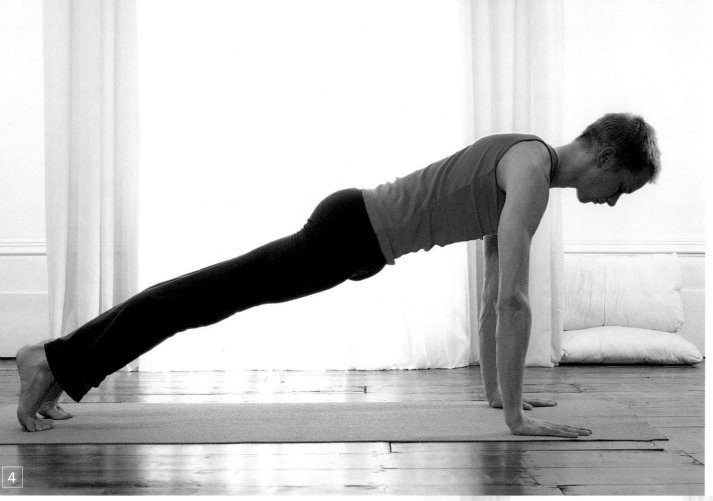

4

Step 4
Walk hands backwards until they are directly under shoulders.

Step 5
Exhale as you flex arms to lower hips in line with whole body, then **inhale** as you extend arms again. Repeat 5 times.
Flex spine upwards, **exhale**, then walk hands back to feet as you **inhale**. **Exhale** to roll back up to standing.

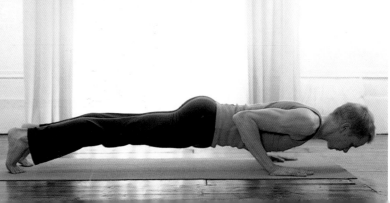

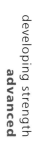

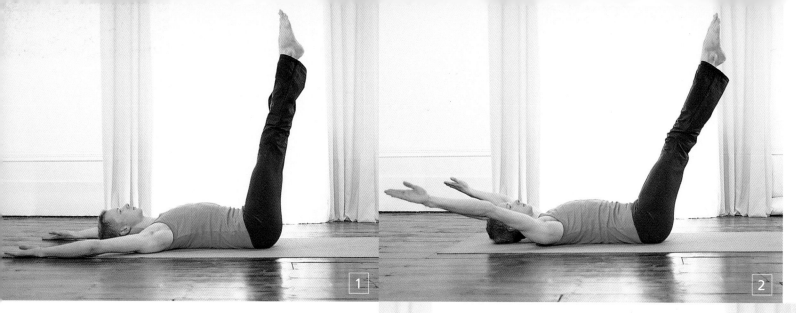

Step 2
Lower legs to 45 degrees, contracting abdominals. **Inhale** to begin raising arms.

Step 1
Lie face up with both legs lifted directly in line with hips, arms stretched overhead.

Step 3
Reach arms towards feet, lifting upper body from floor as if floating.

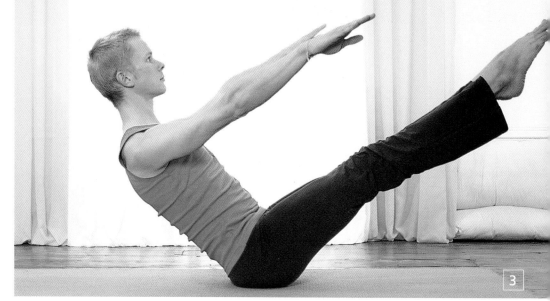

teaser to develop a deep strength of the abdominals, balance and control of the torso in an unsupported posture

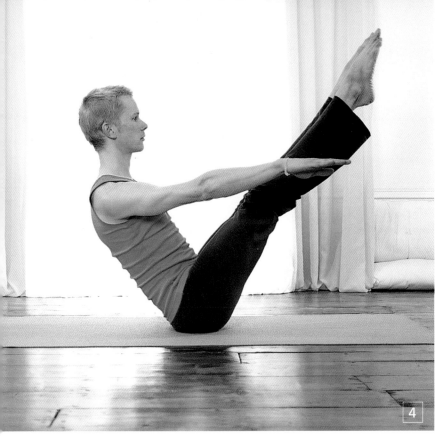

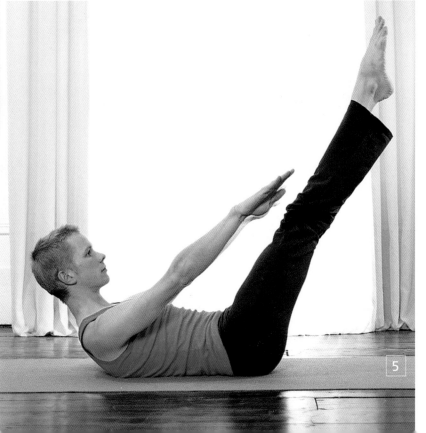

Step 4
Maintain V position with weight through sacrum.

Step 5
Exhale to roll down, one vertebra at a time, contracting buttocks, and return to start position.

note The teaser is one of the most challenging exercises, so progress slowly and do only a few repetitions until your strength develops.

developing strength **advanced**

99

Step 1
Lie face up with pelvis in neutral, abdominals contracted, legs extended. **Inhale**, contract inner thighs and buttocks, raise legs to vertical, directly over hips.

Step 2
Extend legs over head, rolling onto lower shoulder blades as you **exhale**.

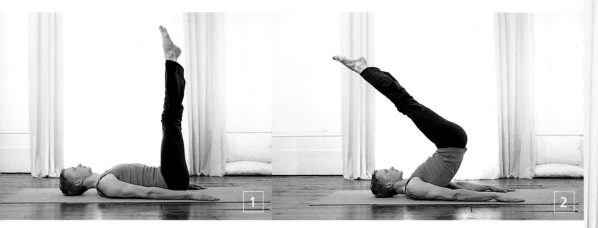

note

If you have moderate to severe symptoms of the cervical spine, avoid this exercise.

Step 3
Inhale to extend legs upwards, pressing into arms until legs approach vertical. **Exhale** to roll down slowly one vertebra at a time, using power of deep abdominals to control movement so both sides of pelvis make contact with floor evenly. Lower legs to start position.

jack knife

to develop strength of the deep abdominals, buttocks and thighs, and release of the shoulders and upper spine

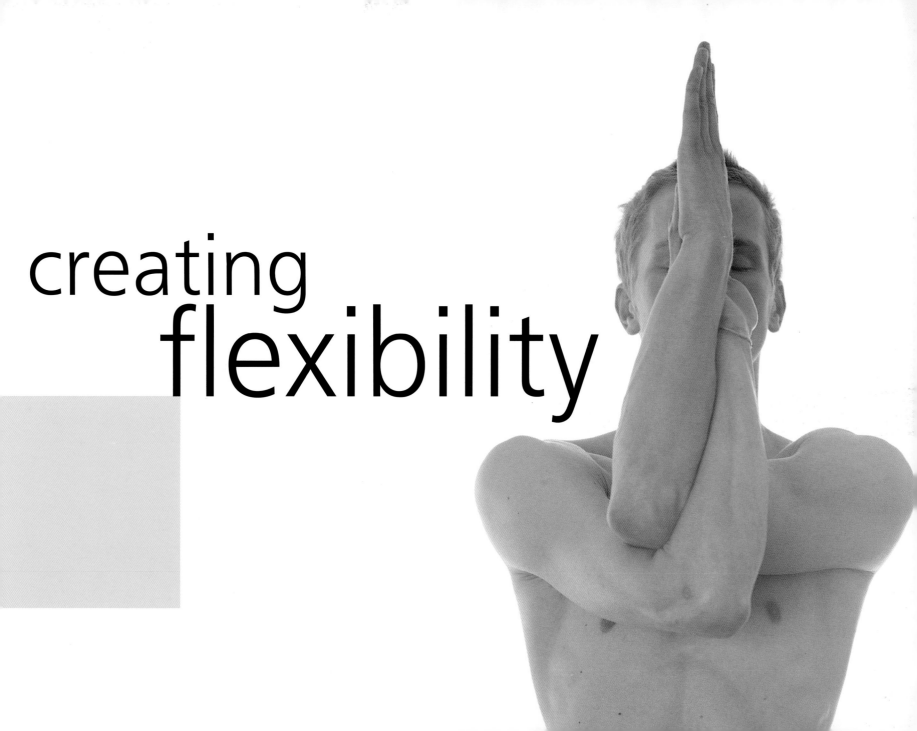

creating
flexibility

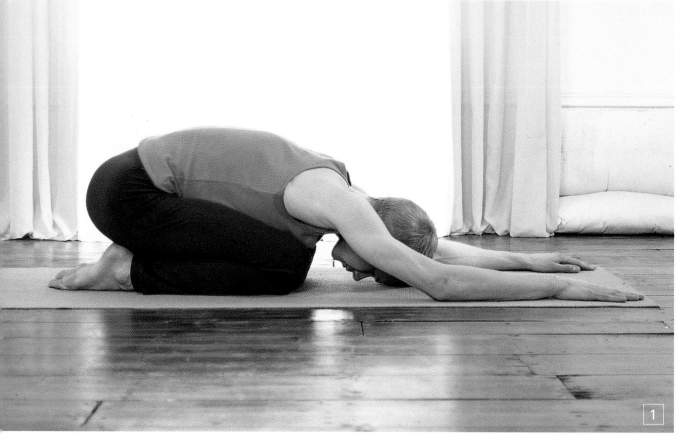

Step 1
Elongate spine, increasing distance between pelvis and head, and stretch through arms to release shoulder blades from ribcage. Also move into the posture to release spine between exercises, especially after extension movements.

note

The posture can also be used to develop a sense of breathing into the posterior ribs to improve rib mobility and motion of the thoracic spine.

creating flexibility

spine release position

to elongate the spine, to mobilize the shoulder blades on the ribcage and to release the spine between different exercises

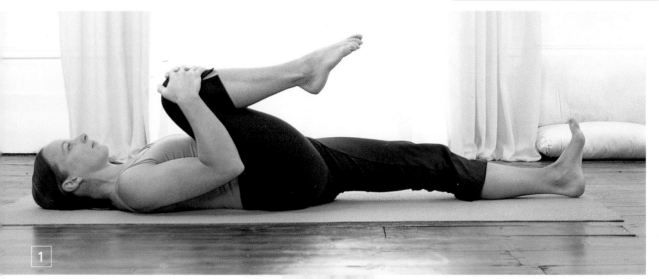

Step 1
Lie face up, knees flexed, feet hip-distance apart, pelvis neutral, shoulders released.
Flex right knee to chest, lengthening left leg with ankle flexed and press through heel to increase sense of lengthening, maintain neutral pelvis and release of lower spine.

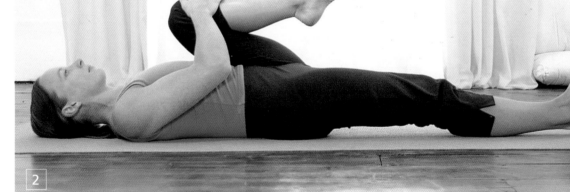

Step 2
Return to start position.
Repeat on other side.

hip and lumbar stretch to improve flexibility of the hips and lumbar spine

creating flexibility

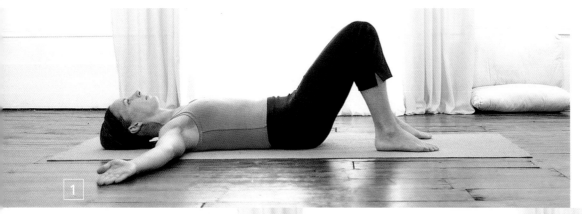

Step 1
Lie face up with arms extended outwards, palms up, legs hip-distance apart, knees flexed.

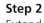

Step 2
Extend left leg to floor, lower right leg to left, placing right foot under left knee.

Step 3
Rotate face to right, lengthening both arms away from torso, then reach left arm across chest. Return to start position. Repeat on other side.

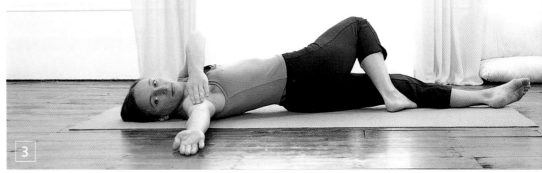

creating flexibility

torso and spine stretch to increase flexibility of torso and spine

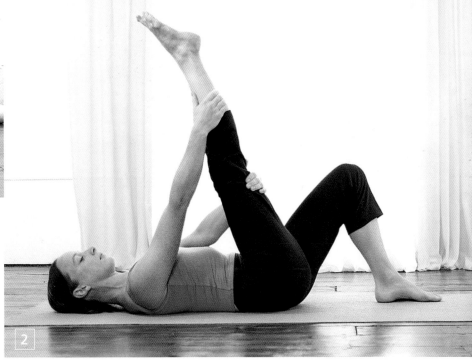

Step 1
Lie with legs hip-distance apart, knees flexed, pelvis neutral, shoulders released.

Step 2
Lengthen right leg upwards, placing hands around knee and calf.

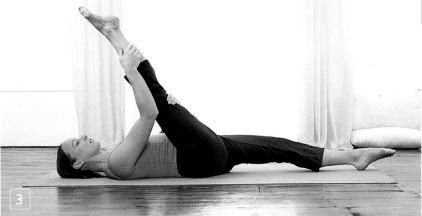

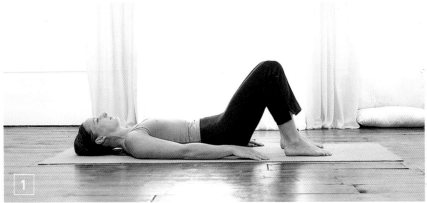

Step 3
Maintain pelvis in neutral, elongating leg towards torso while releasing upper body. Slowly lengthen left leg to floor to increase stretch.
Return to start position.
Repeat on other side.

Variation
Use a towel around your foot to assist in extending leg.

isolated hamstring stretch to increase flexibility of the hamstrings

creating flexibility

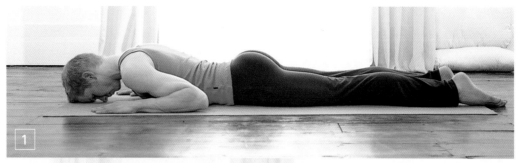

Step 1
Lie face down, abdominals contracted, legs extended, feet together, hands placed flat on either side of head.

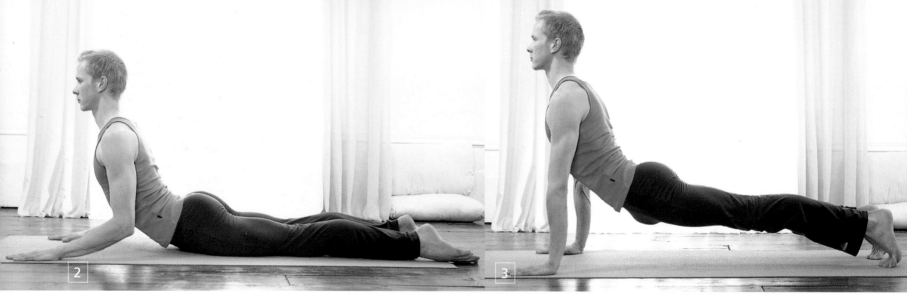

Step 2
Press into palms, lengthening arms and extending torso.
Maintaining pelvis in contact with floor, contract buttocks and thighs.

Step 3
Extend torso, maintaining pelvis in neutral, until torso is elevated and weight is through toes and balls of feet and upper body.
Return to start position.

creating flexibility

chest/abdominal stretch to increase flexibility of the chest

Step 1
Stand with spine lengthened, pelvis neutral, abdominals contracted, shoulders released, feet in parallel and hip-distance apart.

Step 2
Step forward with right leg into lunge position, right knee directly above right ankle, maintain neutral pelvis. Extend arms upwards.

Step 3
Lower left knee to floor. Return to standing position. Repeat on other side.

psoas stretch to increase flexibility of the hip muscles

creating flexibility

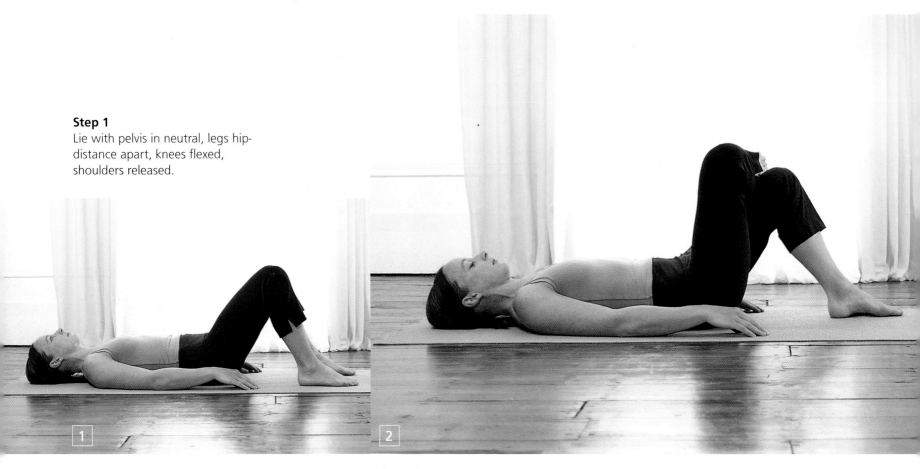

Step 1
Lie with pelvis in neutral, legs hip-distance apart, knees flexed, shoulders released.

Step 2
Cross right leg over left thigh, opening right hip outwards.

piriformis stretch

to reduce muscular tension in the deep buttock muscles, realign the sacro-iliac joint and release the lumbar spine

Step 3

Place hands around left thigh, maintaining left leg at right angle to floor, pelvis neutral. Draw left leg towards chest using power of upper back, and deepen stretch.

Step 4

Return to start position.
Repeat Step 2 with left leg over right thigh.

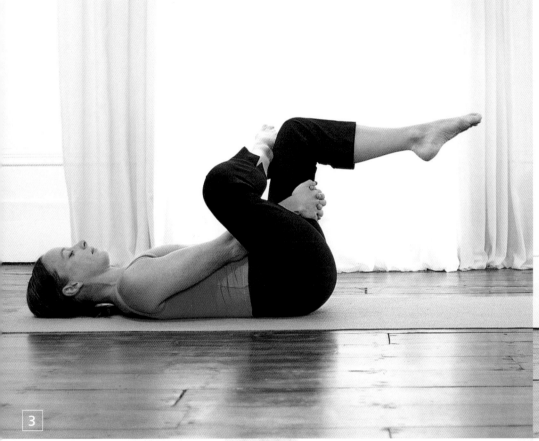

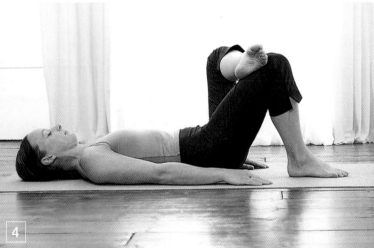

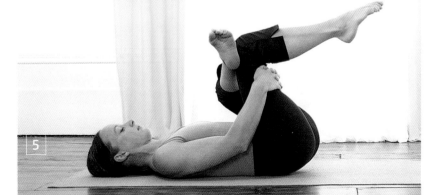

Step 5

Place hands around right thigh, maintaining right leg at right angle to floor, pelvis neutral.
Draw right leg towards chest using power of upper back, and deepen stretch.

creating flexibility

109

Step 1
Place hands directly under shoulders and knees under hips, maintaining lower spine in neutral. **Inhale**.

Step 2
Exhale, contracting abdominals to spine, flexing spine, tucking chin towards chest.

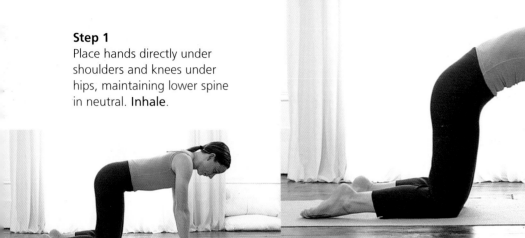

Step 3
Return to start position on **inhalation**.

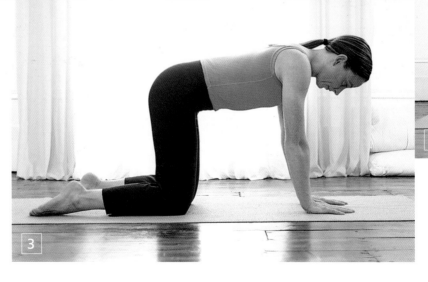

Step 4
As you **exhale**, allow spine to extend, contract buttocks, draw shoulder blades down ribs, gently extend neck, looking upwards. Return to start position.

creating flexibility

cat to facilitate spinal awareness and mobility of the spine and pelvis

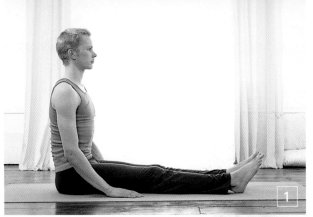

Step 1
Sit with spine lengthened, weight even through pelvis, legs extended in parallel, shoulders released.

note

Sense your breath reaching into the back of the torso, and send the breath to the base of the spine to release and lengthen the lumbar spine.

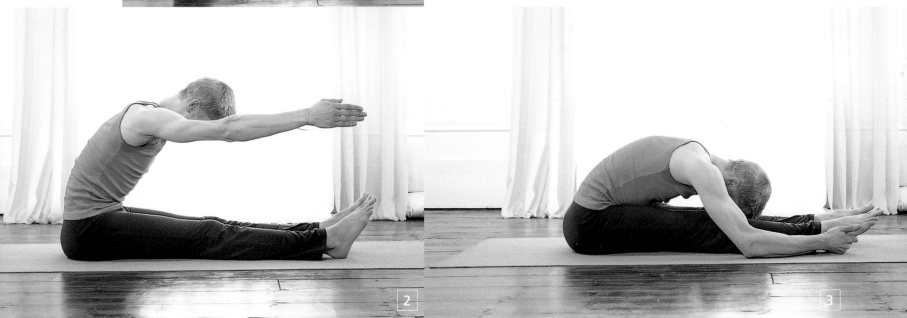

Step 2
Extend spine upwards from pelvis, stretching arms towards ankles.

Step 3
Flex spine, bring torso towards legs, press knees into floor, flex ankles. Return to start position.

spine and hamstring stretch to increase flexibility of the spine and the hamstrings

creating flexibility

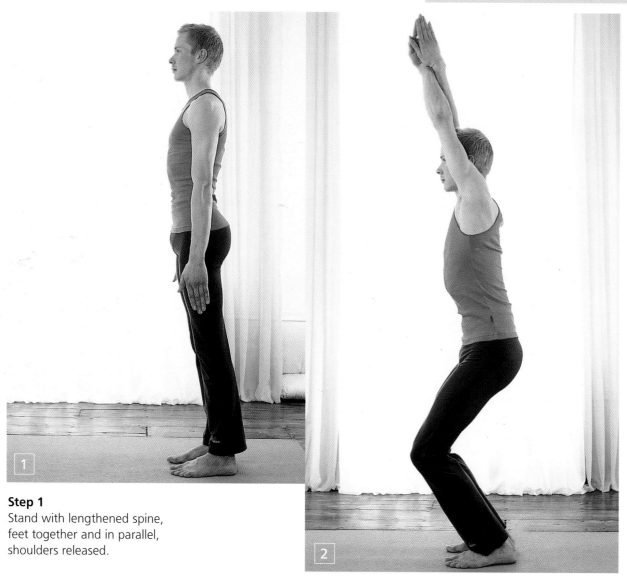

Step 2
Elongate arms over head and cross
wrists, contract abdominals.
Flex knees bringing thighs parallel
to floor, extend mid-spine lifting
chest, maintain contact of
heels on floor.
Return to start position.

Variation
Stand with spine resting against
a wall.

Step 1
Stand with lengthened spine,
feet together and in parallel,
shoulders released.

creating flexibility

shoulder/upper torso stretch to increase flexibility of the upper torso

112

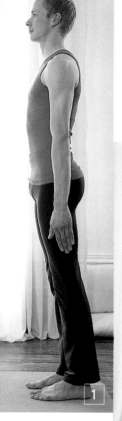

Step 1
Stand with feet hip-distance apart, lengthen spine, release lower spine, contract abdominals.

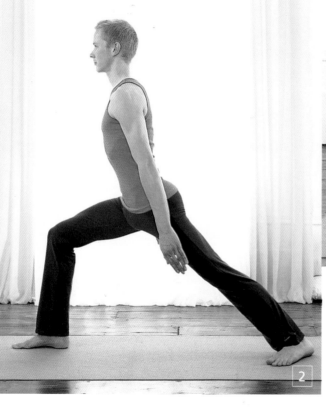

Step 2
Flex right knee in line with ankle, lengthen spine, maintaining pelvis in neutral, extend left leg backwards.

Step 3
Position right hand on floor slightly in front of right foot, open chest, rotate spine, place left hand on pelvis, look upwards. Return to standing position. Repeat on other side.

trunk and hip flexor stretch
to strengthen and tone the legs and facilitate flexibility of the hips and torso

creating flexibility

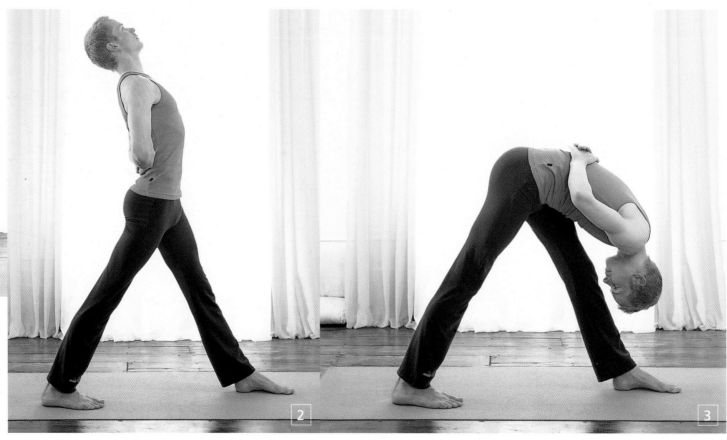

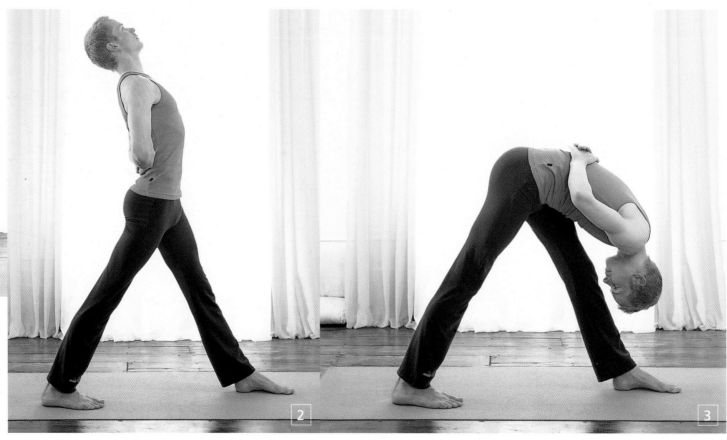

Step 1
Stand with spine lengthened, abdominals contracted.

Step 2
Place arms behind mid-spine, holding forearms, open chest. Step forward with left leg, extending spine, maintaining neutral pelvis.

Step 3
Flex spine, lengthening torso downwards to left knee, maintaining extension of legs. Return to start position. Repeat on other side.

creating flexibility

114

spine and pectoral stretch to increase the flexibility of the spine and chest

specialized
programmes

These specialized programmes have been designed to emphasize specific areas to allow you to focus on developing strength, balance, coordination and flexibility. Use the same number of repetitions as given for each individual exercise.

pelvic tilt **page 49**

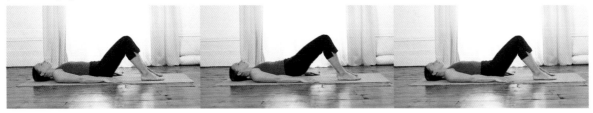

spine twist **page 51**

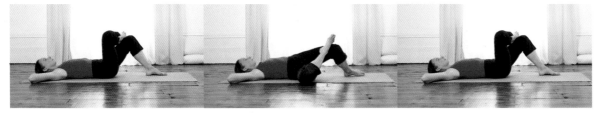

pelvic isometric **page 52**

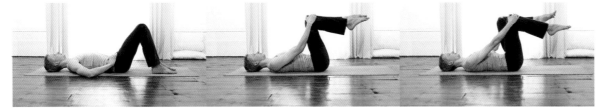

abdominal curl **page 54**

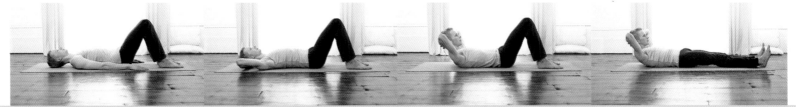

lumbo-pelvic programme
to strengthen, stabilize and improve functional movement of the lumbar spine and pelvic region, and for prevention of and recovery from injury

bridge **page 56**

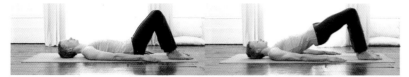

clam **page 57**

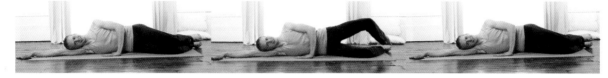

spine extension **page 59**

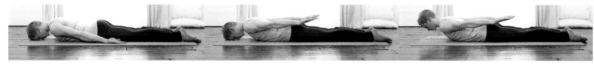

spine stretch forward **preliminary** **page 64**

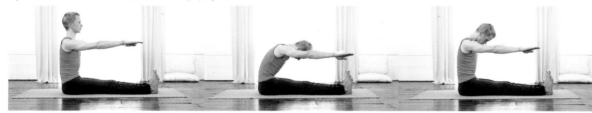

side leg lift **preliminary** **page 65**

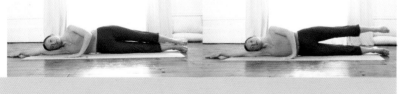

single leg kick **preliminary page 66**

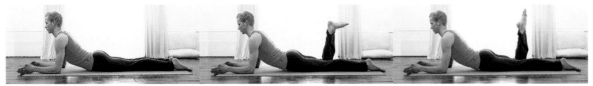

roll over **advanced page 79**

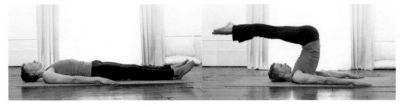

swimming **advanced page 88**

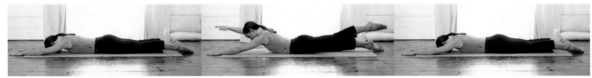

hip and lumbar stretch **page 103**

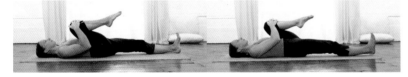

torso and spine stretch **page 104**

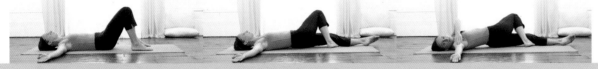

lumbo-pelvic programme (continued)

isolated hamstring stretch **page 105**

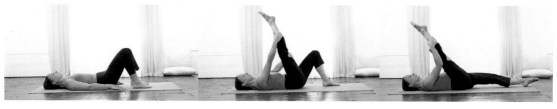

psoas stretch **page 107**

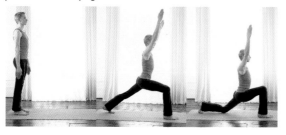

cat **page 110**

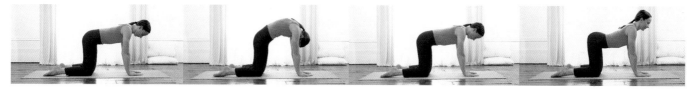

spine and hamstring stretch **page 111**

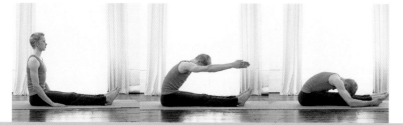

spine and pectoral stretch **page 114**

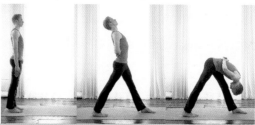

arm lift **page 47**

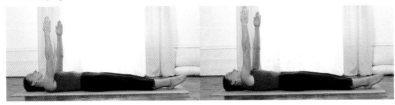

floating arms **page 48**

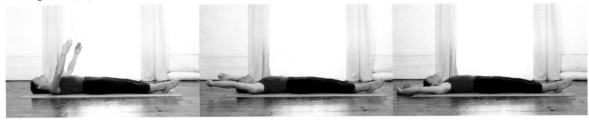

cervical curl **page 53**

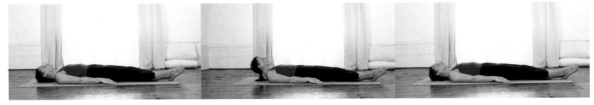

cobra **page 58**

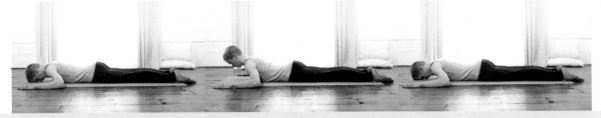

shoulder girdle/upper torso programme
to release, stabilize and protect the neck from overuse and misuse, and to strengthen the upper torso
and facilitate its coordinated function

roll up preparation **page 60**

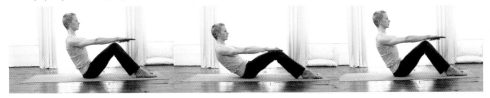

spine stretch forward **preliminary** **page 64**

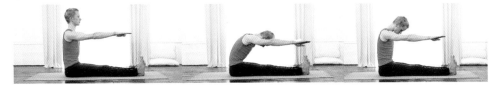

rowing **intermediate** **page 70**

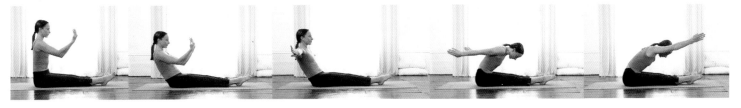

roll up **advanced** **page 76**

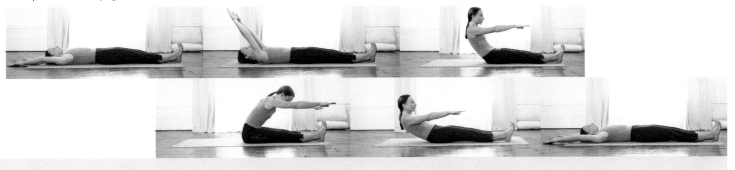

breast stroke **advanced** **page 86**

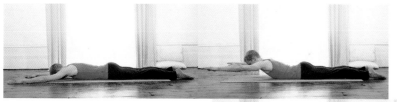

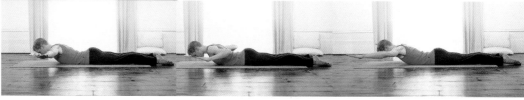

boomerang **advanced** **page 94**

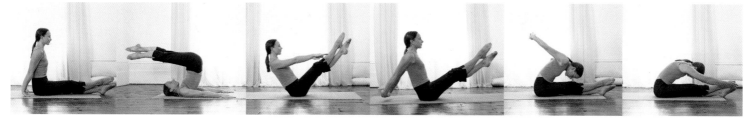

push up **advanced** **page 96**

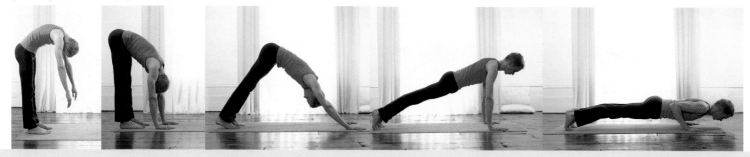

shoulder girdle/upper torso programme (continued)

spine release **page 102**

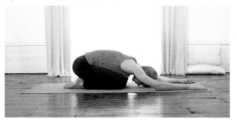

cat **page 110**

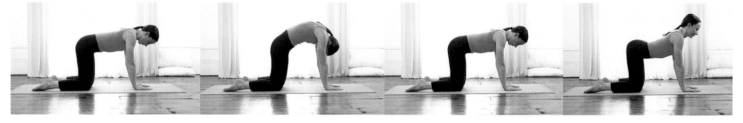

shoulder/upper torso stretch **page 112**

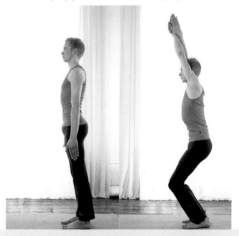

spine and pectoral stretch **page 114**

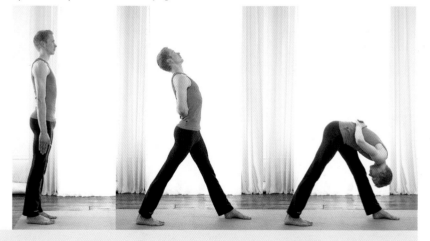

glossary

abdominals or 'abs' is the popular name for the rectus abdominus muscle that runs vertically down the entire front of the abdomen. It supports the abdominal organs and draws the front of the pelvis upwards.

anterior at or towards the front.

articulate to form a joint. The vertebrae articulate with the intervertebral discs.

extension straightening.

flexion bending.

gluteals or gluteus maximus – the muscles that form the buttocks.

intervertebral between the vertebrae.

lateral to the side or sideways.

lordosis forward curvature (of the cervical or lumbar spine).

lumbo-pelvic relating to the small of the back, made up of the lumbar vertebrae, the sacrum, the hip bones and the coccyx.

obliques the internal and external obliques are muscles in the abdomen. The internal oblique crosses the abdomen horizontally, compresses the abdomen and moves the torso. The external oblique is a side muscle of the abdomen. It compresses the abdomen and is used when moving the torso in any direction.

piriformis a muscle that acts on the hip joint. It pulls the thigh out sideways when the hip is bent and turns the thigh outwards when the hip is extended.

posterior at the back of or behind something.

sacro-iliac (joints) the two joints in the lower back where the sacrum meets the ilia (part of the hip bone).

scapula the shoulder blade.

thoracic relating to the thorax, which is the part of the body enclosed by the ribcage.

vertebral body the main part of each vertebra. It is the vertebral bodies that are linked together to form the spinal column.

zygapophyseal joints or facet joints, formed by the articular processes on the left and right sides of the vertebra. They hold the intervertebral joints in place.

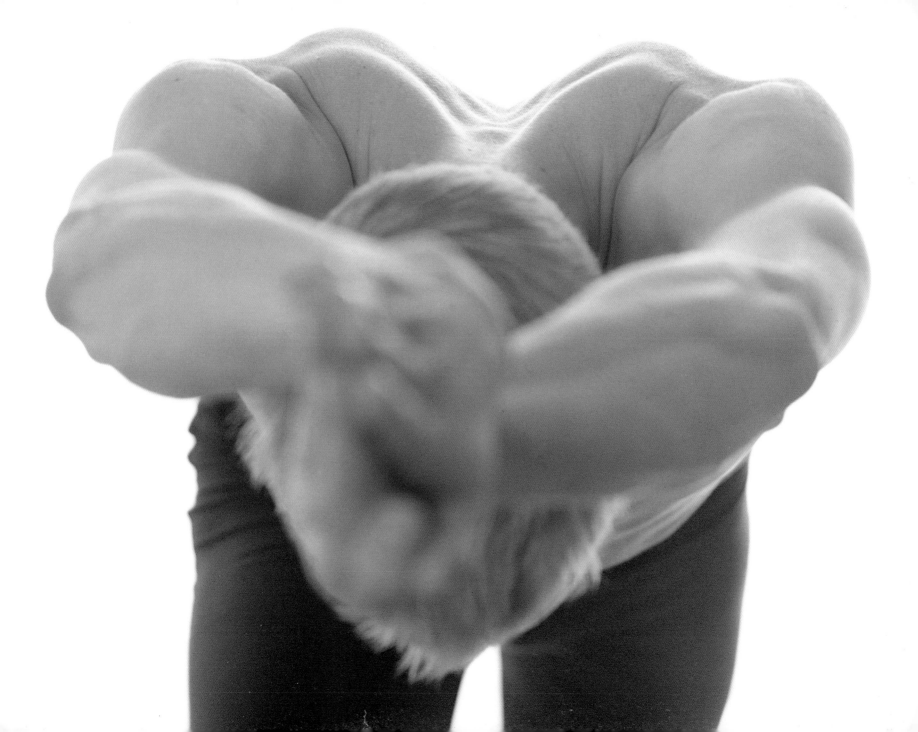

index

abdominals
abdominal curl, 54
chest/abdominal stretch, 106
corkscrew, 80
double leg stretch, 69
hip twist, 81
jack knife, 100
neck pull, 84–5
oblique twist, 78
roll up, 76–7
roll up preparation, 60
rowing, 70–1
single leg stretch, 63
teaser, 98–9
the V, 67
age, 40
alignment, 11, 42
arms
arm lift, 47
floating arms, 48
leg pull down, 92
leg pull up, 93
push up, 96–7
rowing, 70–1

balance
kneeling side kick, 90
side bend, 91
teaser, 98–9
boomerang, 94–5
breast stroke, 86–7
breathing, 11, 38–9, 44
bridge, 56
shoulder bridge, 82–3

buttocks
bridge, 56
clam, 57
double leg kick, 74–5
jack knife, 100
piriformis stretch, 108–9
shoulder bridge, 82–3

cat, 110
centring, 11
cervical region, 18
cervical curl, 53
see also neck
chest, 19
chest/abdominal stretch, 106
cobra, 58
push up, 96–7
spine and pectoral stretch, 114
clam, 57
clothing, 38
cobra, 58
coccyx, 19
concentration, 11
coordination, 11
corkscrew, 80

discs, intervertebral, 20

endurance, 11

fitness levels, 40
flexibility, 36–7, 101–14
floating arms, 48
flowing movements, 11

fluids, drinking, 39

hamstrings
bridge, 56
isolated hamstring stretch, 105
push up, 96–7
shoulder bridge, 82–3
single leg kick, 66
spine and hamstring stretch, 111
spine stretch forward, 64
hips
corkscrew, 80
hip and lumbar stretch, 103
hip twist, 81
kneeling side kick, 90
psoas stretch, 107
single leg circle, 62
trunk and hip flexor stretch, 113
working in turnout, 45
the hundred, 68

imaging, 11
injuries, 26
integration, 11
intervertebral discs, 20
isolated hamstring stretch, 105

jack knife, 100
joints, spinal, 20

knee lift, 50
kneeling side kick, 90

legs
clam, 57
double leg kick, 74–5
double leg stretch, 69
isolated hamstring stretch, 105
jack knife, 100
knee lift, 50
kneeling side kick, 90
leg extension, 55
leg pull down, 92
leg pull up, 93
open leg rocker, 73
push up, 96–7
shoulder bridge, 82–3
side leg lift, 65
single leg circle, 62
single leg kick, 66
single leg stretch, 63
spine and hamstring stretch, 111
spine stretch forward, 64
trunk and hip flexor stretch, 113
the V, 67
working in turnout, 45
ligaments, 20, 28
listening to your body, 35
lordosis, lumbar, 21
lumbar spine, 19
bridge, 56
corkscrew, 80
hip and lumbar stretch, 103
hip twist, 81
injuries, 26
lumbar lordosis, 21
lumbo-pelvic programme, 37, 116–19

movement, 22–3
pelvic isometric, 52
pelvic tilt, 49
piriformis stretch, 108–9
shoulder bridge, 82–3
single leg circle, 62
spine extension, 59
stability, 28

mat work, 15
medical conditions, 39–40
muscles, 24–5, 28, 30–1, 37
music, 38

neck
    cervical curl, 53
    neck pull, 84–5
    releasing, 44–5
    shoulder girdle/upper torso
        programme, 120–3
nervous system, 31
neutral pelvis, 42
nutrition, 39

oblique twist, 78

pain, 39
pelvic floor exercises, 45
pelvis
    cat, 110
    lumbo-pelvic programme, 37, 116–19
    neutral pelvis, 42
    pelvic isometric, 52
    pelvic tilt, 49

piriformis stretch, 108–9
practising, 35
preparation for exercises, 34–5
psoas stretch, 107
push up, 96–7

relaxation, 11
ribs, 44
roll over, 79
roll up, 76–7
    preparation, 60
rolling like a ball, 72
rowing, 70–1

sacral region, 19
sacro-iliac joints, 19
    pelvic isometric, 52
    piriformis stretch, 108–9
scapular stabilization, 43
shoulder girdle
    breast stroke, 86–7
    cobra, 58
    jack knife, 100
    roll up, 76–7
    shoulder bridge, 82–3
    shoulder girdle/upper torso
        programme, 37, 120–3
    shoulder/upper torso stretch,
        112
    spine release position, 102
side bend, 91
specialized programmes, 115–23
spine
    anatomy, 18–21

looking after, 26–7
    stability, 28–31
spine and hamstring stretch, 111
spine and pectoral stretch, 114
spine extension, 59
spine release position, 102
spine stretch forward, 64
spine twist, 51
strength, 36, 61–100
studio work, 15
swimming, 88–9

teaser, 98–9
thighs
    working in turnout, 45
    see also legs
thoracic spine, 19
    cobra, 58
torso and spine stretch, 104
transversus and multifidus
    co-contraction, 42–3, 55
trunk and hip flexor stretch, 113
turnout, 45

the V, 67
vertebrae, 18
vertebral canal, 21

water, drinking, 39

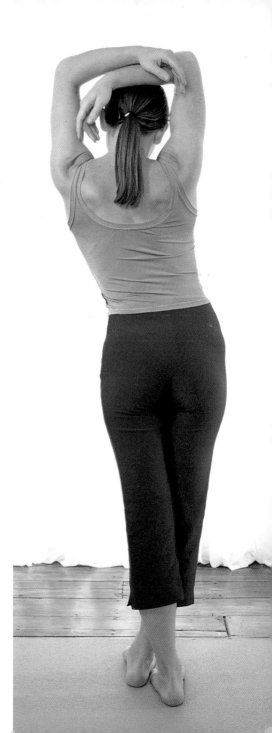

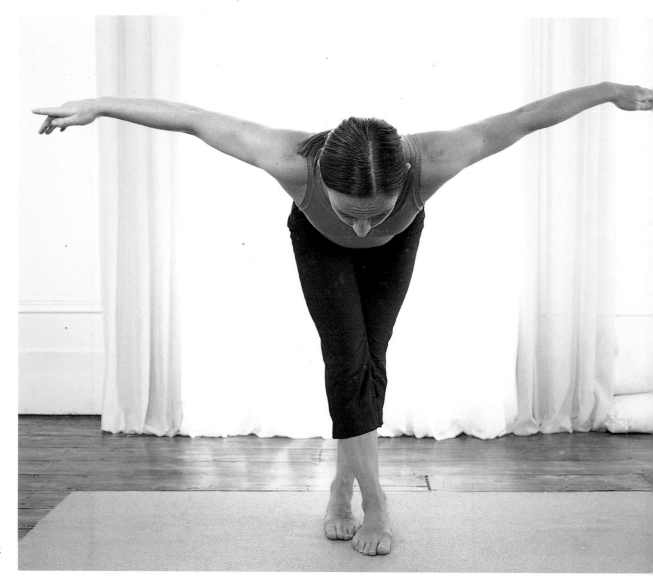

Executive Editor **Anna Southgate**
Editor **Sharon Ashman**
Senior Designer **Rozelle Bentheim**
Designers **Maggie Town** and **Bev Price**
Production Controller **Edward Carter**
Photographer **Niki Sianni**
Illustrations **Bounford.com**
Models **Briany Plant, David McCormick**
and **Robert Clarke**

acknowledgements